Other books in the 10 Best Questions® series
by Dede Bonner, Ph.D.

The 10 Best Questions® for Surviving Breast Cancer
The 10 Best Questions® for Living with Alzheimer's
The 10 Best Questions® for Recovering from a Heart Attack

The 10 Best
QUESTIONS®

for *Living with Fibromyalgia*

The Script You Need
to Take Control of Your Health

DEDE BONNER, PH.D.

Foreword by Dr. Patrick B. Wood

A FIRESIDE BOOK
PUBLISHED BY SIMON & SCHUSTER
NEW YORK   LONDON   TORONTO   SYDNEY

NOTE: Dr. Dede Bonner and 10 Best Questions, LLC, own the registered trademarks the 10 Best Questions®, the 10 Worst Questions™, and The Magic Question™.

Fireside
A Division of Simon & Schuster, Inc.
1230 Avenue of the Americas
New York, NY 10020

First Fireside trade paperback edition September 2009

FIRESIDE and colophon are registered trademarks of Simon & Schuster, Inc.

For information about special discounts for bulk purchases, please contact Simon & Schuster Special Sales at 1-800-456-6798 or business@simonandschuster.com.

The Simon & Schuster Speakers Bureau can bring authors to your live event. For more information or to book an event contact the Simon & Schuster Speakers Bureau at 1-866-248-3049 or visit our website at www.simonspeakers.com.

Manufactured in the United States of America

10 9 8 7 6 5 4 3 2

Library of Congress Cataloging-in-Publication Data
Bonner, Dede.
   The 10 best questions for living with fibromyalgia : the script you need to take control of your health / by Dede Bonner.
      p. cm.
   "A Fireside book."
   Included bibliographical references and index.
   1. Fibromyalgia—Popular works. 2. Fibromyalgia—Miscellanea. I. Title. II. Title: The ten best questions for living with fibromyalgia.
   RC927.3.B66 2009
   616.7'4—dc22   2009020048

ISBN 978-1-4165-6053-1
ISBN 978-1-4165-6088-3 (ebook)

This book is dedicated to my graduate business students at Curtin University of Technology in Perth, Western Australia, The George Washington University in Washington, D.C., and Marymount University in Arlington, Virginia, who have inspired and taught me through their Best Questions.

Acknowledgments

I would like to thank the following people who made this book possible: my devoted husband, Randy Bonner; my loving mother, Jane Anderson; my brilliant editor at Simon & Schuster, Michelle Howry; Jessica Roth, my publicist; my literary agent, Paul Fedorko of the Trident Media Group; former Simon & Schuster CEO, Jack Romanos; editor-in-chief of Touchstone Fireside, Trish Todd; my attorneys, Lisa E. Davis of Frankfurt Kurnit Klein & Selz, PC, and Ellen W. Stiefler of the Stiefler Law Group, PC, all of whom believed in me and in my vision for the 10 Best Questions® series.

I'd also like to thank the sixty experts I interviewed for this book for graciously sharing their time and expertise and for reviewing my drafts. I send my special thanks to Dr. Patrick Wood for contributing the foreword.

Thanks to my university colleagues, Dr. John P. Fry, Dr. Donald G. Roberts, and Dr. Virginia Bianco-Mathis of Marymount University in Arlington, Virginia; Dr. Cynthia Roman and Dr. Elizabeth B. Davis of The George Washington University in

Washington, D.C.; and Dr. Margaret Nowak, Dr. Robert Evans, and Dr. Alison Preston of Curtin University of Technology in Perth, Western Australia.

Lastly, I want to thank all of my graduate business students in the United States and Australia for their enthusiasm, research efforts, and best questions. I'd especially like to thank the following students who researched related topics as their class projects and the experts they interviewed.

From Curtin University of Technology: Muna Abdullah Al-Raisi, Felicite Black, Russell Byrne, Linda Deutsch, Stephen Dunstan, John Gourlay, Cheryl Hayward, Ashley Hunt, Brad Kelly, Mark Latham, Erika Lozano, Carmen Ng, Sharin Ruba, Cheree Schneider, Balwant Singh, John Stopp, Jennifer Talbot, Alan Thornton, Anne VanDenElzen, John Wareing, and Peter Westlund.

From Marymount University: Arend Fish, Jaime Boyer, Kelly Foster, Jennifer Hanley, Shannon Hiltner, Michelle Ray, and George Straubs.

Contents

Foreword

---

by Dr. Patrick B. Wood

These are exciting times for those of us whose lives are touched by fibromyalgia, whether as persons affected by the disorder, patient advocates, health-care providers, or researchers whose careers are dedicated to advancing scientific insight. In the last thirty years, our understanding of the disorder has expanded dramatically. In the early days of the disease, fibromyalgia was seen as either a musculoskeletal disorder affecting the muscles and soft tissues, or else a psychiatric disorder in which negative emotions were somehow transformed into painful bodily sensations.

There is now, however, convincing evidence that the symptoms that characterize fibromyalgia—pain, stiffness, sleep disturbances—stem from changes within the central nervous system, i.e., the brain and spinal cord. As a result of these insights, approaches to the assessment and treatment of the disorder have likewise undergone rapid transformation. The recent approval by the U.S. Food and Drug Administration (FDA) of drugs specifically for the treatment of fibromyalgia and the establishment of guidelines for patient assessment and treatment bear witness—the times indeed are a-changing.

Yet, while the science of fibromyalgia is rapidly advancing, there remains an unfortunate lag between these insights and the level of care available to affected individuals at the community level. Indeed, as you may have experienced, the approach to fibromyalgia by clinicians varies widely—from those who see their role in diagnosis and management as an essential aspect of routine patient care, to those who dismiss the reality of the disorder out of hand. This, in part, is why the book you are holding in your hands represents a valuable asset, because it can help to empower you to make better decisions regarding the partners you choose in your personal journey toward wellness.

Given the choice, you would naturally want to work with professionals who are both knowledgeable about fibromyalgia and compassionate in their approach to those affected by it. If you live in a large community containing a variety of health-care providers, Dr. Bonner's insights can help you to select who your best doctor might be. On the other hand, if your choices are more limited, whether by finances or the size of your community, this book can help you make the most of your situation by helping to improve your ability to care for yourself and by helping to foster better relationships with your current providers.

As someone who has provided health care to literally hundreds of people affected by the disorder, I have come to appreciate that difficulties in communication between fibromyalgia patients and their health-care providers represent one of the greatest challenges to optimal clinical outcomes. While fibromyalgia is defined by the presence of chronic widespread pain, in reality it is a complex disorder that affects multiple bodily systems, including one's cognitive abilities. The term *fibro fog* is often used to describe the impact of fibromyalgia on a person's ability to think and concentrate, which ranks among the most troubling but least appreciated aspects of the disorder by many clinicians.

The mismatch between a clinician's potential understanding of the disorder (i.e., as a form of muscle pain) and the broad spectrum of symptoms associated with it (including cognitive problems) is perhaps to blame for the friction that characterizes the relationship between fibromyalgia patients and their doctors. (Imagine the perspective of the provider left wondering why it is that so many of his or her patients with muscle pain are so difficult to communicate with!) Insights regarding changes in brain function may help to explain why fibromyalgia patients are affected by fibro fog—insights that will, I expect, eventually become a routine part of the clinical management of the disorder.

In the meantime, the principles embodied in this book can help you to overcome the challenges that fibro fog represent by enabling better organization of your thoughts prior to each clinic visit—by prioritizing problems, outlining important questions, using memory aids to help employ medical decisions following the visit—which will, in turn, help you make the most of your visit. There is also sound advice to help you better manage other complex issues beyond the clinical visit, including making informed choices regarding patient support groups, navigating the world of complementary and alternative treatments—even managing finances.

Let's face it: There are a lot of books out there on living with fibromyalgia that range in quality from the truly helpful to well . . . good for wrapping fish in. When I was first asked to write the medical foreword for the book you have in your hands, I have to admit that I was just a bit skeptical at first. Would the average patient really benefit from (yet another) fibromyalgia book added to their collection? In this case, the answer is a heartfelt *yes*! In the classroom of life's lessons for fibromyalgia patients, let's consider this one required reading.

Dr. Patrick B. Wood *is a respected authority on the cause and treatment of Fibromyalgia Syndrome who has been twice recognized by the National Institutes for Health for his innovative research. Dr. Wood is Assistant Professor in the Departments of Family Medicine, Psychiatry and Anesthesiology at Louisiana State University Health Sciences Center in Shreveport, where he directs both the Fibromyalgia Research Program and the Fibromyalgia Care Clinic. He is a nationally known speaker on the subject of fibromyalgia and has presented his work at scientific conferences around the world.*

Introduction

———

The most important questions are often the ones you didn't know to ask. Even the best doctors in the world can't give you the right answers unless you ask them the right questions first.

But how do you know what the right questions are? "Ask your doctor." You've heard it a million times, but do you *really* know what to ask? What if you don't know very much about fibromyalgia yet, feel intimidated by your doctor's expertise, or just simply feel overwhelmed by your diagnosis?

More than ten years ago when my mother suffered a major heart attack, I felt overwhelmed. As I nervously watched her vital sign monitors bounce around, it occurred to me that I didn't know what to ask the doctors about her condition. In that moment of total helplessness, the only thing I had was questions. But I just didn't know what to ask.

I vowed to learn how to ask better questions. When I started taking my mom to her follow-up doctor appointments, I spent time researching her medical options and planning questions for her doctor. I wanted to be a well-informed consumer for her sake so that I could make sure she was getting the very best care possible.

This experience sparked my interest in questioning skills. As I read about questions, I was surprised to learn how little attention most people pay to them. It seems that our society is so focused on solutions and answers that we rarely stop to consider the quality of our questions.

I started teaching questioning skills as part of my graduate-level business classes in Washington, D.C., and Perth, Australia. My students liked it so much that I developed the concept of "The 10 Best Questions" as a way for them to learn questioning skills, team dynamics, and research skills all at once. Since 2003, I've taught hundreds of students who have interviewed thousands of experts. For example, my students have researched what to ask when you buy a house, get married, adopt a dog, hire a financial planner, change careers, invest in stocks, retire, plan a wedding, talk to your teenagers, choose a university, and want to have a great sex life.

I conducted a series of interviews with top question askers to learn their secrets. Helen Thomas, the legendary White House reporter, is famous for her press conference questions to every president since John F. Kennedy. She told me, "Before a news conference I would think, What's the best question to ask? I have the courage of ignorance in my questions. I always get nervous, figuring out what to ask a president. But I believe you have to be curious and keep asking why."

Dorothy Leeds, who has authored nine books on questioning skills, told me, "Everything in my life has come about from asking questions, every major change. It's amazing how questions can enrich your life, both from a career and personal stand-point."

Peter Block, an international management consultant and the author of the book *The Answer to How Is Yes,* said, "There's a deeper meaning to asking questions. It's a stance you take in the world, a desire to make contact and get connected."

I talked with many professional interviewers like Susan Sikora, a TV talk show host in San Francisco; Debbie Nigro, a New York radio host; and Richard Koonce, a journalist and consultant in Brookline, Massachusetts. Each responded with a version of, "You are only as good as the questions you ask." Since then, I've focused my consulting work on helping CEOs and organizations develop their own Best Questions.

For the information specific to this book, I interviewed two former U.S. surgeons general and the president of the National Fibromyalgia Association. I talked with prominent experts in fibromyalgia diagnosis and treatments, sleep hygiene, nutrition, exercise, preventive health, stress, fitness, special populations, smoking and alcohol cessation, and personal, family, and sexual relationships. I also interviewed "everyday people" with fibromyalgia, including Martha Beck, a best-selling author, life coach, and columnist for *O, The Oprah Magazine*, and Rosie Hamlin, best known for her famous 1960s hit song, "Angel Baby."

So, what are the traits of the best question askers? They are smart, curious, and fearless, yet humble enough to learn from someone else. They value listening and inquiry. Great question askers see every person they meet as a walking encyclopedia of valuable information just waiting to be unlocked by the right questions. And finally, as Albert Einstein once said, "The difference between me and everyone else is my ability to ask the right questions."

The 10 Best Questions in this book won't make you an instant Einstein. And as the Question Doctor, I certainly don't claim any Einstein-like brilliance. I believe that a good mind knows the right answers, but a great mind knows the right questions. Now that great mind is yours. This is a book "for smarties," not for dummies.

Each list of The 10 Best Questions is derived from as many as nine hundred questions from hundreds of sources, including books, journals, worldwide print media, Web sites, and expert interviews. A Best Question has to really earn its title of "Best." I've also included the "best answers" my experts and research provided so you'll know when you are hearing the full story. The information in this book should not replace medical guidance or professional counseling.

There is one more question per chapter that I call "The Magic Question™." A Magic Question is that one great question that even smart people rarely think to ask—a gut-level question you usually think of when it's too late.

In writing this book, I've taken a practical and holistic approach to fibromyalgia to make you an empowered patient. I want to help with your key decisions, choices, and relationships by suggesting what you can ask your doctors, medical experts, partner, family, friends, and ultimately yourself after a diagnosis of fibromyalgia.

Your lifetime prescription for good health is to stay informed. As former surgeon general Dr. C. Everett Koop told me in an interview, "There's nothing that will lead to better medical care than a knowledgeable patient."

The 10 Best Questions in this book give you the actual script in hand for each major conversation and decision you are facing. Be sure to ask plenty of your own questions, too. Question guru

Helen Thomas says, "There's no such thing as a bad question, only a lot of bad answers."

As the Question Doctor, I sincerely hope the following Best Questions will ease your journey and give you the courage to take charge of your own health. Your doctor may be an authority on medicine, but you are the world's foremost expert on yourself.

PART I:

Talking with Your Doctor

Two common concerns expressed by people who have been diagnosed with fibromyalgia are fear of the unknown and fear of not communicating well with their doctors. Your doctors can help you make decisions, but you have to ask the right questions first.

Many people are intimidated by their doctors' knowledge and are reluctant to ask them questions. Former acting U.S. surgeon general rear admiral Dr. Kenneth P. Moritsugu comments, "For the older generation, the relationship is that the doctor knows everything and you just accept what the doctor has to say."

But patient-physician relationships are changing. The president of the National Fibromyalgia Association, Lynne Matallana says, "The number one most important thing people with fibromyalgia can do is to effectively communicate with their healthcare providers. Some patients have a reputation for being difficult, but you won't be difficult if you go to your appointments well prepared to ask the right questions."

Use this book to help you. This is no time to be shy, worry about hurting the doctor's feelings, or be secretly afraid that he or she may not "like you" if you ask questions. There's no reason to be aggressive in asking your questions but be firm with your doctor that you expect answers.

To be heard, you may need to repeat your questions or concerns. According to a 1999 study published in *The Journal of the American Medical Association* (*JAMA*), when patients are trying to talk, doctors typically interrupt after just twenty-three seconds.

Persist through interruptions. If your doctor interrupts you before you make your point, try saying, "I'd like to finish" or, "Can we come back to my concerns later?"

This book is primarily for people who have been diagnosed with fibromyalgia but will also be valuable if you have a related disease, like chronic pain syndrome, or suspect you might have fibromyalgia.

The Best Questions in the first chapter suggest what to ask your doctor when you are first getting your diagnosis. Use chapters 2, 3, and 4 to find a great doctor who is "fibro-friendly" and knowledgeable. If you want a second opinion, ask the Best Questions in chapter 5.

Take chapter 6 with you to the doctor's office when you are going for regular wellness checkups. Chapter 7 covers the special concerns for men with fibromyalgia.

This book isn't necessarily meant to be read from cover to cover but rather to be grabbed and consulted for each crossroads and conversation in your journey with fibromyalgia. Remember that even the best doctors in the world can't give you the right answers if you don't ask the right questions first.

CHAPTER 1: THE 10 BEST QUESTIONS

About Your Diagnosis of Fibromyalgia

> First the doctor told me the good news: I was going to
> have a disease named after me.
>
> —Steve Martin

I hurt all over." That's the cry of an estimated 3 to 15 million Americans who are afflicted with fibromyalgia, a poorly understood chronic pain disorder characterized by widespread aches, stiffness, multiple tender points, fatigue, and sleep disturbances. Other common symptoms include depression, difficulty concentrating, numbness or tingling sensations, heightened sensitivity to light and noise, and anxiety.

Fibromyalgia affects mainly women of all ethnic groups, but it can occur in men and children as well. Due to its often debilitating nature, patients' family members and friends are also affected. Many people with fibromyalgia have difficulty fully functioning in their daily lives, including working and raising children.

Millions of people with fibromyalgia have been misdiagnosed with a dizzying list of other ailments. Many doctors are still unfamiliar or hostile to fibromyalgia as a "real disease." Dr. Kim Dupree Jones, a fibromyalgia expert at the Oregon Health & Science University explains, "The average patient sees five or six doctors over seven to eight years to get an accurate diagnosis. People with this diagnosis can be much maligned. They are often told that it's all in their heads."

Martha Beck, well-known fibromyalgia patient, life coach, and best-selling author, recalls, "My twelve years of being in constant pain also had the awful social ramifications of being in constant pain that no one understands. You are told you are a wimp and that you are making it up, that you're lazy, that you're hysterical. That was just hell on wheels."

Confronting a diagnosis like fibromyalgia can be frightening and confusing.

These following Best Questions are ones you may not think to ask your doctor, along with notes on why they're important and the "best answers." The assumption here is that you've recently been diagnosed with fibromyalgia and are discussing your case with either a primary care physician or a specialist.

THE QUESTION DOCTOR SAYS:

Don't ever hesitate to ask other questions that are not in this book. There truly are no dumb questions, especially for a diagnosis like fibromyalgia. Don't be afraid to ask the doctor to repeat anything you don't understand. Be politely insistent about getting answers to your questions. This is your body and you deserve to have a well-educated mind inside of it.

GOOD ADVICE FROM THE PRESIDENT OF THE NATIONAL FIBROMYALGIA ASSOCIATION

Lynne Matallana says, "It's really important that you bring an advocate with you to doctor appointments, especially in the beginning, because many people with fibromyalgia have 'fibro fog.' Sometimes it's very difficult to remember what the doctor says. Your advocate can ask questions and take notes for you."

⟩⟩⟩THE 10 BEST QUESTIONS
About Your Diagnosis of Fibromyalgia

1. How do you know for sure that I have fibromyalgia?

This question may be the most important question you ever ask in your life.

Many people never think to ask this question. They are too shocked, confused, or relieved to finally have a label for their mysterious ailments. But fibromyalgia is a complex illness without a definitive diagnostic test, as compared to reading a mammogram or analyzing a laboratory blood sample.

In order to be diagnosed with fibromyalgia, a patient must meet two criteria: 1) three or more consecutive months of pain occurring above and below the waistline and on the left and right side of the body (chronic widespread pain); and 2) significant tenderness in at least eleven of the eighteen tender points on light palpation (defined as 4 kilograms of pressure). See the tender point diagram at the National Fibromyalgia Association's Web site: http://www .fmaware.org/site/News2?page=NewsArticle&id=6263.

The tender point exam is the *only* diagnostic test for fibromyalgia and is considered to be 80 percent accurate. It was formally established by the American College of Rheumatology (ACR) in 1990. But doctors' skills vary in how much pressure they apply during the test and how to interpret the results. This is especially true of doctors who are unfamiliar with or hostile to fibromyalgia.

Keep in mind that fibromyalgia diagnoses are wrong 20 percent of the time. Many of the symptoms of fibromyalgia mimic those of other diseases, such as hypothyroidism, polymyalgia rheumatica, neuropathies, lupus, multiple sclerosis, and rheumatoid arthritis. Make sure you've had all the appropriate tests and examinations to rule out other possible disorders. With fibromyalgia as the newest medical buzzword, your doctor may be tempted to label you too quickly. Similarly, some doctors misdiagnose lesser known types of dementia as the high profile Alzheimer's disease.

Remember that you aren't challenging your doctor's wisdom or credentials. A good doctor welcomes questions and believes you have every right to know as much as possible about your fibromyalgia.

As fibromyalgia expert Dr. Michael McNett says, "Easily half of the doctors out there don't believe that fibromyalgia exists. The patient should learn what the ACR criteria are. That's the answer. Be educated about the eighteen tender point spots around your body." The bottom line is, don't jump on the "fibromyalgia train" unless you really have a ticket.

THE QUESTION DOCTOR SAYS:

Be sure to phrase this question, "How sure . . ." rather than "Are you sure. . . ." When you ask a yes/no question like "Are you sure?" you won't get as much information from your doctor as you will when you phrase it in a more open-ended way, like "How sure . . . ?"

---

2. What caused my fibromyalgia? What is my prognosis?

In reality, your doctor is not likely to know the answers, but it's only human nature to ask these questions. No one really understands yet what causes fibromyalgia. Theories range widely from trauma-induced causes to chemical imbalances and autoimmune functions.

Your **prognosis** is your long-term health outlook. Fibromyalgia is not a terminal illness (you won't die from it), but it is

chronic (there is no known cure). The intensity of your symptoms may vary, but they probably will never disappear. Many people live full lives with their fibromyalgia in remission for long stretches of time.

Fibromyalgia sufferer, Rosie Hamlin, songwriter and the lead singer of the 1960s hit song, "Angel Baby," recalls, "My doctor told me that I wasn't going to die from my fibromyalgia, even though I thought I was."

A good follow-up question is, "Are my children, siblings, and other blood relatives at risk for fibromyalgia?" While most people with fibromyalgia don't have relatives with it, there is a genetic component that researchers are just now starting to untangle.

3. What are my best treatment options?

Currently, there are several prescription medications for pain management, more drugs for sleep disorders, and other drugs for related symptoms, like irritable bowel syndrome. See chapter 8 for a comprehensive discussion on medications.

In the absence of any surefire medication, you are wise to work with your doctor to develop a multifaceted treatment plan. As chapter 9 explains, there are many treatments broadly called **complementary and alternative medicine (CAM)** that may help you. Two of the most common CAM treatments, massage therapy and acupuncture, are discussed in chapters 12 and 13.

Most fibromyalgia patients benefit from sleep management therapies. See more in chapter 14.

4. What lifestyle changes can I make that will help my overall health and comfort?

Making a **lifestyle change** means modifying or eliminating long-held habits in order to adopt and maintain new healthier habits.

Your doctor will most likely address weight management, diet, and physical activity or exercise.

To improve your diet and weight, ask yourself the Best Questions in chapter 16. There are also practical Best Questions to ask your doctor about weight management in chapter 6.

A regular program of gentle exercise will help you to maintain muscle tone, reduce pain, and manage flare-ups. See more advice in chapters 17 and 18 on exercise and finding a great gym and personal trainer to help you meet your fitness goals.

Adopting healthy lifestyle changes is a very sensible approach for managing fibromyalgia. A healthy lifestyle can also literally save your life by preventing a heart attack, stroke, or the onset of Type 2 diabetes.

5. What can I do to avoid flare-ups? How can I manage my depression, anxiety, and/or stress?

Triggers for fibromyalgia flare-ups vary widely and often can't be anticipated. Many people do find, however, that it helps to systematically avoid certain circumstances, foods, smoking, or stressors, and to find relief for their sleep disturbances.

Negative emotions can be a heavy (but understandable) burden for many fibromyalgia patients. This is especially true if you've spent months or years getting an accurate diagnosis, living with severe pain, and having little or no support from your loved ones.

Your doctor may prescribe medications for you or suggest various CAM therapies. To proactively take charge of your health, see the Best Questions in chapter 19 on emotions, on better relationships with your partner (chapter 20), on intimate relations (chapter 21), with children (chapter 22), and with other people (chapter 23).

Don't hesitate to seek professional help. Chapters 2, 3, and 4 can help you find a competent psychologist or counselor.

6. What can I do about my fibro fog?

Fibro fog or **brain fog** is a common symptom of fibromyalgia. Patients experience cognitive dysfunction, such as impaired concentration, memory problems, inability to multitask, diminished attention span and mental speed, and related depression, anxiety, and disturbed sleep symptoms. Hearing from your doctor about medications or lifestyle changes to fight fibro fog will help you get over thinking you are losing your mind or intelligence.

Don't downplay or overlook your fibro fog. Dr. Patrick Wood, a fibromyalgia expert in Seattle, says, "I have so many patients tell me, 'I can live with the pain. The fatigue is hard. But the worst thing about fibromyalgia is that I can't think straight. I can't make a living.'"

7. What other medical conditions do I have or could I develop that should be treated or monitored?

This question covers two scenarios: 1) overlapping conditions with fibromyalgia, and 2) other illnesses you may have or develop independent of fibromyalgia. Overlapping conditions include myofascial pain syndrome (chronic muscle pain), temporomandibular joint jaw pain (TMJ), irritable bowel syndrome (IBS), chronic fatigue syndrome (CFS), painful menstrual periods called endometriosis, and depression. Assuming your doctor is knowledgeable about fibromyalgia and has done a complete medical history and exam on you, ask how your other ailments might be related to fibromyalgia and about appropriate treatments.

In the second scenario, both you and your doctor should stay alert to any existing, new, or potential non-fibromyalgia diseases.

For example, don't let your fibromyalgia overshadow the diagnosis and treatment of heart disease, diabetes, or allergies. See more in chapter 6 on wellness checkups.

8. What advice do you have for me about my ability to continue working? For applying for disability assistance?

Your fibromyalgia symptoms may be preventing you from performing well on the job or being there at all. If this is true for you, make sure you tell your doctor and ask for her advice and medical assistance. Your financial future and quality of life are at risk.

Likewise, if you face possible disability, you'll first need the medical facts from your doctor. Getting disability assistance from the Social Security Administration is not easy and often takes a great deal of time and perseverance. This is a potentially complex discussion that you may need to have several times with your doctor. Get more details on disability at the National Fibromyalgia Association's Web site, www.fmaware.org/site/PageServer?page name=topics_disability.

9. What advice do you have for me about pregnancy and/or menopause?

You may not have considered how pregnancy or menopause could affect your fibromyalgia. The interaction of fibromyalgia and hormones is only beginning to be understood. But researchers have found correlations between fibromyalgia and pregnancy complications, reduced fertility, and troublesome menopausal symptoms.

Some women experience a drop-off in fibromyalgia symptoms during pregnancy, while others suffer more. Pregnancy is possible with fibromyalgia, but symptom management may require a little extra help and advice from your doctor.

Likewise, fibromyalgia patients' response to menopause also varies widely. Discuss your personal situation with your doctor, such as breastfeeding concerns after pregnancy or taking hormone replacement therapy (HRT) after menopause.

10. What symptoms are serious enough that I should call you? How often should I see you on a regular basis?

Asking these questions now just makes good sense so you'll know when and how frequently to contact your doctor.

If you are contemplating seeing a specialist, ask either: "Where do you recommend that I be treated?" or "Do you have a fibromyalgia specialist you can refer me to?" See chapter 2 on referrals.

THE QUESTION DOCTOR SAYS:

Take a recording device to your appointments and ask your doctor's permission to record his answers. There will be a lot of new information coming at you. Good doctors won't mind and will actually appreciate your desire to be an active player in your health care.

❭ The Magic Question

What is the most hopeful thing you can tell me about my diagnosis?

Try to think of your diagnosis as more hopeful than helpless. At least you may feel relieved to finally know your symptoms have a name and there are millions of other sufferers. You and your invisible illness have been vindicated. You aren't crazy after all.

As fibromyalgia expert and patient advocate, Devin J. Starlanyl, says, "Validation is a very important issue because this is an invisible illness. People with fibromyalgia often don't get the support they need because a lot of people, including physicians, think it's all in the mind."

Fibromyalgia as a medical disorder has finally gained respect and interest. This means there are now megadollars for research on fibromyalgia drugs, therapies, origins, and understanding its causes and potential cure. Ideally, researchers will soon find new ways to precisely tailor highly individualized treatment plans.

So, ask your doctor for your good news, too. What's the best outcome you've seen in cases like mine? It will help to put things into perspective. You deserve some good news today, too.

CONCLUSION

There is nothing more comforting or empowering than being a well-informed patient. Being an empowered patient means you are involved as an active player along with your doctors in understanding and treating your fibromyalgia. Get the good habits of a healthy lifestyle and a questioning mind now in your battle against fibromyalgia.

THE 10 BEST RESOURCES

American College of Rheumatology. "Fibromyalgia." http://www .rheumatology.org/public/factsheets_original/fibromya_new.asp.

FibroCenter. "How Your Health Care Professional Diagnoses Fibromyalgia." www.fibrocenter.com/images/FM_Diagnosing.pdf.

Fibromyalgia Information Foundation. "Home." www.myalgia.com/ index.html.

Fibromyalgia Network. "Symptoms." http://fmnetnews.com/basics -symptoms.php.

Matallana, Lynne, and Laurence A. Bradley. *The Complete Idiot's Guide to Fibromyalgia,* 2nd ed. New York: Penguin Group, 2009.

Mayo Clinic. "Fibromyalgia Symptoms or Not? Understand the Fibromyalgia Diagnosis Process." www.mayoclinic.com/health/fibromyalgia-symptoms/ AR00054.

National Fibromyalgia Association. "Diagnosis." www.fmaware.org/site/ PageServer?pagename=topics_diagnosis.

National Institute of Arthritis and Musculoskeletal and Skin Diseases. "Fibromyalgia: Questions and Answers About Fibromyalgia." www .niams.nih.gov/Health_Info/Fibromyalgia/default.asp.

Ostalecki, Sharon. *Fibromyalgia: The Complete Guide from Medical Experts and Patients.* Boston: Jones and Bartlett Publishers, 2007.

Trock, David H., and Frances Chamberlain. *Healing Fibromyalgia.* Hoboken, NJ: John Wiley & Sons, 2007.

CHAPTER 2: THE 10 BEST QUESTIONS

To Get a Reliable Referral for the Best Doctor

> The competent physician makes himself acquainted not
> only with the disease, but also with the habits and
> constitution of the sick man.
>
> —Cicero

Because fibromyalgia is a chronic (long-term) disorder, you will need ongoing medical care from your primary care physician or several specialists. Even if you choose to stay with your primary care physician, you are likely to need at least one specialist, such as a specialist in sleep disorders or pain management. See the list of specialists in chapter 3.

Regardless of the type of doctor you see, it's very important to find a "fibro-friendly" one whom you can trust as a long-term partner. Not all doctors, even rheumatologists, believe that fibromyalgia is a real condition with real pain. Lynne Matallana, the president and cofounder of the National Fibromyalgia Association, went to thirty-seven doctors before she got a correct diagnosis in 1995. Now she says, "It's so important to find a doctor and ask questions to make sure this is a doctor worthy of you going to see."

Dr. Michael McNett, a fibromyalgia expert, explains, "There are still many, many doctors who aren't onboard with fibromyalgia and believe it's an excuse that women have made up so they can sit around and feel sorry for themselves. There are many negative ideas about fibromyalgia out there, but it used to be much worse."

Over and over again, people with fibromyalgia say, "I want a doctor who really listens to me and respects me as an individual." This level of support and communication with your doctor is precious. You want to know you are receiving top quality care, the latest treatments, and up-to-date knowledge on research.

Check the National Fibromyalgia Association's Web site (www.fmaware.org) for its "fibro-friendly" doctor list by location. You can also find a specialist by asking your primary care physician, or through family members, friends, coworkers, or a local fibromyalgia support group.

If you are like most people, when you have a conversation about getting a referral to a new doctor, you'll probably only ask for the name, address, and phone number. Perhaps you'll ask, "Do you like this doctor?" or "Where is he located?" Most likely, you trust the person giving you the referral.

In blind faith, you call the prospective doctor's office and schedule the first appointment you can get. As you hang up, you feel a rush of relief because the doctor's receptionist wasn't from Mars and you could get in to see this new doctor quickly.

But you may have just jumped headfirst into potentially dangerous quicksand—and don't even know it. Here's why. It may not have occurred to you that you know virtually nothing about this new doctor. Okay, perhaps you did an Internet search, but you have already let your most important ally and information source slip away—the person who already knows him and gave you this referral.

Stop and think about this for just a moment. Here you are on the brink of establishing a very important new relationship with the person who will ultimately hold your health and well-being in his hands. This doctor's judgment and experience will be absolutely critical at every step of the way.

Maybe you feel shy about questioning your current doctor closely about his referral, fearful you will somehow insult his judgment. Maybe you secretly worry your current doctor will think you are dumb or too aggressive if you ask more questions.

Get over it. This is a very important referral and you have every right to know the qualifications of the doctors treating you.

There are hundreds of potential reasons behind the referral, ranging from the two of them are Friday night poker pals to being long-time professional partners. The point is that you just don't know until you ask.

This chapter will help you find a reliable best doctor who is willing to work with you. The following list of 10 Best Questions includes questions to ask in two scenarios. In the first situation, use questions 1 and 2 and the Magic Question when talking with someone with medical expertise.

In the second situation, you are getting the referral from current patients, friends, or family members—your peers. When talking with nonmedical people, ask all ten questions below and the Magic Question. As you start, be sure to find out first if this prospective doctor honors your medical insurance and takes new patients.

Don't hesitate to ask. So much is at stake. Having a top doctor with a deep knowledge of fibromyalgia and a sympathetic outlook will make a huge difference in your care.

In chapter 3, you'll talk directly to this new doctor. But for now, don't skip this important preliminary step of getting a quality referral.

>>> THE 10 BEST QUESTIONS
To Get a Reliable Referral for the Best Doctor

1. Why are you recommending this doctor?

One of the best ways to judge a prospective doctor's quality is through the recommendation from another doctor. Most doctors are sincerely interested in the well-being of their patients and refer them to the doctors they believe offer the best care.

If you are asking a medical professional this question, listen for an answer that includes how impressive this doctor is in his field. Key phrases are "participated in clinical trials" and "presented papers at professional conferences." These are extra-effort activities that earn respect among medical peers.

But don't stop there. Listen for clues about this prospective doctor's bedside manner as well as his superstar performance at last year's medical conference.

Some doctors fall into referral patterns of always recommending the same doctor down the hallway or a former college roommate. While this isn't necessarily a bad thing, it helps if you know this piece of background information.

If you are talking with other patients or friends, a good follow-up question is, "How did you originally find this doctor?" For example, if the person found this doctor without doing her homework, or even worse, from the Yellow Pages, take this person's diminished credibility into account as you assess her answers to the other Best Questions.

There are also "insider" Internet sources (see the "good doctor lists" at www.fmaware.org and www.co-cure.org/Good-Doc.htm) but just remember that an online recommendation is not as foolproof as a personal one.

2. How well do you know him or her?

If you are asking a medical professional, you want to hear that this person has worked closely with the recommended doctor for a number of years. If you are seeking a second opinion, the doctors may not know each other as well, so listen for clues about the prospective doctor's reputation.

Don't assume that someone is a good doctor just because your doctor has referred you to him. You may learn they are only social friends, and your doctor has little firsthand knowledge about his friend's real doctoring skills.

If you are asking a current patient, use this question to make sure her judgments aren't based on a short-lived or long-ago relationship.

3. How satisfied are you with this doctor? In your opinion, what are this doctor's strengths and areas that need improvement?

Depending on this person's degree of openness and willingness to talk, you may get all the details you need by simply asking how satisfied she is. Be sure to press gently for details on the areas that need improvement. Everyone has shortcomings. Use this question to decide if you can live with this doctor's particular deficiencies or quirks.

THE QUESTION DOCTOR SAYS:

Be sure to ask open-ended questions. For example, "How satisfied are you?" rather than "Are you satisfied?" A "how" question results in much more valuable information than a question that can have a simple yes/no answer.

4. How well did this doctor communicate with you?

Listen for phrases like:

> I didn't feel rushed when I talked with him.
> He explained everything slowly and used words I could
> understand.
> He acted like he was really listening to me.
> He made me feel comfortable.
> I could finish my sentences without being interrupted.

5. How well has this doctor kept you informed and encouraged you to ask questions?

This bottom-line Best Question cuts to the core of assessing how patient centered this doctor is.

The doctors who are strongly patient centered are more likely to explain treatment options and possible side effects. The best doctors will gladly answer all your questions at any time without exasperation or impatience and will encourage you to learn more about your disease.

A doctor who enjoys giving you full and educational explanations is most likely to treat you with respect. The best doctors encourage questions. In turn, the most knowledgeable patients are usually the most satisfied with their doctors and their care.

6. Did this doctor openly respect your opinions and decisions? Did you ever feel the doctor was talking down to you?

This question helps you to further assess this doctor's attitude and how opinionated he might be when presenting care options. Some people prefer a directive doctor who tells them what to do, whereas others prefer to do their own research and make independent decisions with the doctor's input.

There's no right or wrong way here. Just look for a doctor who is a good match for your own communication style.

7. How well did this doctor support you and your healing process over time?

Your doctor should be your genuine ally in your fight against pain. Asking this question now of a person who has already been through the experience is very important. Her answer will go a long way in helping you to set your expectations for quality care and open communication with this particular doctor.

As Lynne Matallana suggests, "Find out their attitudes about fibromyalgia. Make sure that a doctor's personality or approach is consistent with what you are looking for."

Press gently for more details including how well the doctor handled unexpected complications or advised about lifestyle changes or new treatments. Remember, you want a partner, not just a doctor.

8. When your partner, family members, or friends accompanied you on office visits, did this doctor also include them in the discussions?

This is another question to determine how compassionate and patient centered this doctor is. If he values his patients from a whole-person perspective, it makes sense that the patient's family will be more readily folded into the discussions and decision making.

Good signs are a doctor who looks at everyone in the room when explaining something, asks others if they have questions, and encourages taking notes or making tape recordings of the meeting.

9. How accessible was this doctor or office staff after hours or on short notice?

Some doctors are generous with their after-hours time, offering you their cell phone numbers or personal e-mail addresses so that you can reach them anytime. Ask the person giving the referral to share any related stories so that you can be realistic about how accessible this doctor will be.

10. How well did this doctor's office staff treat you? Did you ever feel frustrated because of office inefficiency or long wait times to see the doctor?

There's a wide variation in office staff and their responsiveness to patients' needs. You are probably feeling pretty fragile right now, and the last thing you need in your life is a haughty, hostile receptionist or nurse in your doctor's office. You know the one. She acts like it will take an act of divine intervention before she finally agrees to copy a one-page report for your personal files.

You will be depending on this office staff to make sure office appointments are timely, your medical insurance carrier has been properly billed, and your medical records get into all the right hands.

❯ The Magic Question

Do you trust this doctor enough to send your own family to her? Why or why not?

This question works well whether you are asking a doctor or a friend for a referral. Trust is an intangible quality and not something that is easily earned.

Just be aware that the response to this "trust test" question is purely subjective. If you don't fully trust the person you are getting the referral from (think Ms. Yellow Pages), be sure to ask the follow-up question, "Why or why not?"

CONCLUSION

By the time you've asked these Best Questions, you'll have come a long way, baby, from just getting the prospective doctor's name and number.

You'll know so much more about this doctor's background, strengths, shortcomings, philosophy about patient-centered care, communication skills, and what you can expect in terms of ongoing care and office support.

Think of the person making the referral as a "walking encyclopedia" of valuable information about this prospective doctor. These Best Questions are like the key to unlocking his or her personal experiences in a way that will be helpful to you without burdening this person.

Now you are ready to make your first appointment with a new rheumatologist or other fibromyalgia doctor. Don't be tempted to rush past this important preliminary quest for great doctoring. You deserve it. Chapter 3 provides your script for that first visit.

THE 10 BEST RESOURCES

American Medical Association. "Making the Most of an Office Visit." In *American Medical Association Guide to Talking to Your Doctor*. New York: John Wiley & Sons, 2001.

Centers for Medicare and Medicaid. "Choosing a Doctor: A Guide for People with Medicare." http://jobfunctions.bnet.com/whitepaper.aspx ?docid=121268. (Registration required.)

Consumers' Checkbook. "Medical Advice: Is Your Doctor Measuring Up?" www.checkbook.org. (Subscription required.)

Groopman, Jerome. *How Doctors Think.* Boston: Houghton Mifflin, 2007.

HealthGrades. "Research Physicians." www.healthgrades.com. (Charges small fee.)

Manning, Phil R., and Lois DeBakey. *Medicine: Preserving the Passion in the 21st Century,* 2nd ed. Warren, MI.: Springer, 2003.

National Fibromyalgia Association. "The Perfect Fit." http://www.fmaware.org/site/News2?page=NewsArticle&id=5728.

National Institute on Aging. "Talking with Your Doctor: A Guide for Older People." www.nia.nih.gov/HealthInformation/Publications/TalkingWithYourDoctor.

Roizen, Michael F., and Mehmet C. Oz. *YOU: The Smart Patient: An Insider's Handbook for Getting the Best Treatment.* New York: Free Press, 2006.

U.S. News & World Report. "Best Hospitals: Rheumatology." www.usnews.com/directories/hospitals/index_html/specialty+REPRHEU. (Updated annually.)

CHAPTER 3: THE 10 BEST QUESTIONS

For Choosing a Best Doctor

It is a mathematical fact that 50 percent of all doctors graduate in the bottom half of their class.

—Anonymous

Most of us believe that our lives might one day depend on the right decision by a doctor, a belief we have about few other professionals. As you face the realities of living with fibromyalgia that "one day" is no longer abstract. You need Dr. Right—right now.

Before you can proceed, you need to know how to find a best doctor who specializes in fibromyalgia, or at least understands the current medication options and is "fibro-friendly." Having a top doctor can make a world of difference in your treatment, care, and your whole quality of life.

Finding this doctor may seem like a scary and daunting task. Not only do you have a chronic, disabling illness that needs long-term medical care and support, but doctors often misunderstand, disbelieve, or are poorly informed about fibromyalgia symptoms as a "real disease." Asking these Best Questions is your best solution.

When describing their worst experiences with doctors, patients often cite arrogance, dismissive attitudes, and callousness rather than lack of technical expertise, according to a 2006 study at the Mayo Clinic. So not only do you need a technically capable doctor, but also one who will make you feel comfortable and treat you with respect as an active player in your own health care.

In Dr. Jerome Groopman's book, *How Doctors Think,* he says that the attributes of the best doctors are having a relish for knowledge, an insatiable curiosity, pride in their performance, and a "clear, clean joy in sharing with you their knowledge." He cites among the worst attributes a doctor's unwillingness to listen, cynicism, and the tendency to treat all patients the same with "cookie-cutter" or one-size-fits-all treatments.

You may prefer to stay with your family doctor or prefer treatment from a specialist in fibromyalgia. There are no definitive rules for this decision. Some fibromyalgia experts agree with Dr. Daniel Clauw, a pioneer in fibromyalgia research at the University of Michigan, who states, "Rheumatologists are not necessarily any better at treating fibromyalgia than primary care M.D.s."

Even if you prefer to stay with a family doctor for fibromyalgia care, you owe it to yourself to seek a one-time second opinion from a specialist so that you can avoid future regrets or doubts about your diagnosis. See the sidebar list in this chapter on medical specialists. Don't assume that all doctors in these specialties treat fibromyalgia. When you first call a doctor's office, ask the staff if she sees fibromyalgia patients and if your insurance plan is accepted.

The 10 Best Questions in this chapter will help you choose the right person.

THE QUESTION DOCTOR SAYS:

Be sure to tell your doctor at the beginning of your appointment that you have questions and ask when she prefers to answer them. This way you'll know her preference for timing and will have politely informed her that you want enough time to get your questions answered.

Remember that the very best doctors will welcome your questions and your desire to choose a doctor carefully. If a doctor reacts negatively to your questions or refuses to answer them, consider this a red flag. This doctor either has something to hide or may be impatient with you during future office visits. You want an active partnership with your physician, not a "daddy-doctor" relationship with someone who constantly talks down to you.

>>> THE 10 BEST QUESTIONS
For Choosing a Best Doctor

1. Are you board certified? What are your other medical credentials?

Board certification matters.

Board certification assures that the doctor has passed the board requirements for her specialty. In the United States, medical specialty certification is voluntary. Doctors receive their medical licenses after completing medical school and residency requirements. But this doesn't apply to medical specialties like rheumatology, and only sets the minimum competency requirements to treat patients.

The successful completion of the examinations for board certification demonstrates a doctor's exceptional expertise and dedication to a rigorous, voluntary commitment to lifelong learning. This is especially important with fibromyalgia, because of the need to stay current with fast-moving research advances in this field. To maintain board certification, doctors must complete specialty training and periodic exams to demonstrate their ongoing competency. Use the search services of the American Board of Medical Specialties (www.abms.org) to check for a specific doctor's certification.

A valid state license is also very important. Go to the American Medical Association's Web site for links to your state's medical board (www.ama-assn.org/ama/pub/category/2645.html).

Checking on past disciplinary actions and malpractice suits is tougher because most medical professionals don't readily disclose unclean histories. See ChoiceTrust (www.choicetrust.com) or HealthGrades (www.healthgrades.com), two comprehensive Web sites that charge a small fee for their services. Other sources for checking on prior complaints or disciplinary actions are free at Administrators in Medicine (http://docboard.org) and Health Care Choices (www.healthcarechoices.org).

THE QUESTION DOCTOR SAYS:

If you feel shy or intimidated about asking a potential doctor about credentials, ask the office staff, go to the doctor's Web site or bio, or simply do your own search using the resources in this chapter. If you are satisfied about a doctor's credentials, skip asking this question in person.

But don't skip question 1 altogether just because it seems hard to ask. You don't want someone who has served jail time for malpractice prescribing your pain medications!

2. What is your experience with fibromyalgia? How many patients like me have you seen during the past twelve months? Are you comfortable diagnosing and treating people with fibromyalgia?

Experience matters, too—a lot. The number of years of total medical practice is significant, along with the years of specialized practice a doctor has in treating fibromyalgia and related conditions. Keep in mind that fibromyalgia is a relatively "new" syndrome. The condition was first described in the 1880s, named fibromyalgia in 1976, and its diagnostic guidelines (still used today) were established by the American College of Rheumatology in 1990.

It's very important to determine this doctor's prior experience with fibromyalgia and his beliefs about it. Ask this follow-up question: "What percentage of your practice is devoted to treating fibromyalgia and/or chronic pain patients?" The higher the number, the better it is for you.

A good bedside manner can be very comforting, but don't confuse it with competence. A doctor's personality should be your secondary, not the primary, consideration in making your choice. Don't rely on your doctor to be your sole source of hand-holding.

National Fibromyalgia Association's president, Lynne Matallana, offers more advice. "Find out their attitudes about fibromyalgia. Make sure that a doctor's personality or approach is consistent with what you are looking for." There's no sense in seeing a doctor who doesn't want to see you or doesn't believe in fibromyalgia.

3. May I speak to at least one of your patients to see how he or she made out in these same circumstances?

This Best Question was suggested by former surgeon general Dr. C. Everett Koop. He believes it's very important to follow through on patient referrals.

Asking for a referral is more common than you might think. Be sure to follow through and make the phone calls. Chapter 2 gives you specific Best Questions for getting highly reliable referrals.

4. Which hospitals are you affiliated with?

Although people with fibromyalgia generally don't need hospitalization, this answer could be important later. You have two choices: You can choose your doctor first and then go with the hospital where she has admitting privileges. Or you can choose the hospital or fibromyalgia treatment center first and then find a top doctor there. If you live in a rural area or choose not to travel far for treatment, your choices may be more limited.

Ask this follow-up question: "What is the accreditation status of this hospital or medical facility?" See The Joint Commission's Web site (www.jointcommission.org) for more on accreditation.

5. Are you affiliated with any medical schools?

A teaching affiliation with a prestigious medical school is the gold standard when looking for a top doctor. It's a fairly reliable indicator that a doctor is considered by her peers to be a leader in this field. However, it's not a deal breaker, especially for primary care physicians.

The academic doctors who also practice medicine are the most likely to be well informed about the latest research, diagnostic tools, and treatments. This is important to you because new breakthroughs in fibromyalgia treatments are now happening at record pace.

6. Are you involved with any ongoing research projects or clinical trials on fibromyalgia or related diseases?

Experts suggest that you look for doctors who have written about fibromyalgia or related conditions and whose work is often cited in medical journals. If a doctor you are considering has been published, ask for copies of those articles. Even if the articles are written for medical professionals and are very technical, you can learn a lot about this doctor's interests and approach to treating fibromyalgia. Go to PubMed Central (www.pubmedcentral.nih.gov) for a free archive of medical journal abstracts.

7. Are you part of a referral system of medical specialists that I might see for overlapping conditions?

Having fibromyalgia usually means you have other medical problems (called **overlapping conditions**) as well. Ideally, you want to assemble a multidisciplinary medical team including fibromyalgia and sleep specialists, perhaps another doctor for related symptoms, and then such experts as a dietician, personal trainer, acupuncturist, or massage therapist.

At the least you want your primary doctor to be a good team player and communicator. Dr. Brent A. Bauer, director of the Complementary and Integrative Medicine Program at the Mayo Clinic explains, "I think the most important issue is to make sure that all of the care team members are communicating. It's very frustrating when a physician tells a patient one thing, their chiropractor another, and their acupuncturist yet another. Finding providers who are willing to work with you and with each other may take more time, but in the end, the team approach is going to have the greatest chance of success."

Author and fibromyalgia patient advocate Devin Starlanyl advises, "You need to be the coordinator of your medical team." As you see different experts, make sure they are sharing your medical records, test results, and medications history.

8. Do you offer support services and more information about fibromyalgia?

The doctor's answer to this question will indicate if she is patient centered. If you have choices, go to a doctor who emphasizes patient involvement and offers referrals to support services, such as physical therapists, nutritionists, and family counselors.

The best doctors are also good teachers at heart. As former acting surgeon general Dr. Kenneth P. Moritsugu comments, "When the doctor seeks to educate the patient, they are not merely engaging in a two-way conversation. Rather, the doctor is taking it beyond the conversation in order to teach the patient about their medical options and how to take control of his or her own health and well-being."

9. Please describe your preferences for communicating with your patients.

Communication obstacles rank high on patients' lists of complaints. Most people highly value how well a doctor communicates. Just keep in mind that communication is a two-way street, and you can't expect any doctor to just drop everything in response to your calls, questions, or e-mails, especially on a frequent basis.

10. Who covers for you when you aren't available or are on vacation?

This is another question that most patients don't think to ask until they can't reach their doctor when they really need to.

Be sure that your doctor tells you how she will communicate with you if unanticipated problems come up or when she's unavailable or on vacation. Also ask how (calls or e-mails) and when (best times of day) she can be reached.

❯ The Magic Question

What is the last thing you learned about fibromyalgia?

The best answer to this question is not so much what the doctor says but how easily the response rolls off her tongue. If this doctor is truly an excellent doctor and sees plenty of fibromyalgia patients, she'll be able to easily say something like, "Well, I read an article last week" or "I went to a conference last month."

But if she is groping for an answer, look elsewhere. You don't want a doctor who is the last one to know about the newest treatments.

CONCLUSION

If a prospective doctor obviously enjoys—passionately enjoys—the practice of medicine, shows evidence of following new developments in fibromyalgia, thinks hard about you and your problems, asks questions of you, shows a real interest in your answers, and meets the requirements for board certification and experience, you probably have a very good doctor. From the group of good doctors that you find, choose a doctor you can trust and feel comfortable with.

Devin Starlanyl sums up the search for Dr. Right nicely. "Having fibromyalgia is no place for cookbook medicine. If you have a doctor who is a nonbeliever, the best thing you can say to him is, 'Good-bye,' and find someone else to treat you."

WHICH DOCTOR DO I SEE?

The Best Questions in this book work equally well regardless of the type of doctor you are considering. However, due to the nature of fibromyalgia and its overlapping conditions, finding Dr. Right sure can be confusing.

Dr. Kim Dupree Jones, a fibromyalgia expert in Oregon, advises, "Any doctor who has fibromyalgia patients in his practice and has some success in managing them is fine to see. Look for a doctor who is 'fibro-friendly,' has an open mind, will try different medications, and can make good referrals for exercise, behavioral techniques, and dietary help. That's the ideal provider. Also consider nurse practitioners; they are often competent, compassionate healthcare providers for people with fibromyalgia."

Here's a primer on the medical professionals who treat fibromyalgia and pain. You will also want to continue seeing your primary care physician, general practitioner, internist, and/or gynecologist.

> **Rheumatologists** diagnose and treat arthritis and other diseases of the joints, muscles, and bones. Often cited as first-choice fibromyalgia specialists.

> **Pain specialists** are usually board-certified anesthesiologists, neurologists, physiatrists, psychiatrists, and oncologists with additional training in pain management.

> **Neurologists** diagnose and treat nervous system disorders including headaches, back pain, muscle disorders, and fibromyalgia.

> **Orthopedists** specialize in the diagnosis and treatment of bone injuries and muscle and joint problems.

> **Psychologists** diagnose and provide therapy for problems associated with pain, perception, and emotional issues.

Depending on your symptoms, you may also benefit from seeing a sleep expert, psychiatrist, counselor, gastroenterologist (for the digestive system), cognitive behavior therapist (for sleep or other disorders), physiatrist (also called "rehabilitation physician"), naturopath (for supplements), chiropractor, and/or a physical therapist (to restore mobility).

THE 10 BEST RESOURCES

American Academy of Pain Management. "Find An Academy Member Professional." www.aapainmanage.org/search/MemberSearch.php.

American Board of Medical Specialties. "Is Your Doctor Certified?" Board certification for doctors. www.abms.org/wc/login.aspx.

American College of Rheumatology. "Geographic Membership Directory." www.rheumatology.org/directory/geo.asp.

American Medical Association. "DoctorFinder." www.ama-assn.org/aps/amahg.htm. (Search this major database by the state where a doctor practices medicine.)

Consumers Union of U.S. "Doctor, Can We Talk? (How to Develop a Good Relationship with a New Physician.)" *Special Report for Consumer Reports on Health*. July 2001.

Fibromyalgia Network News. "Finding a Quality Physician." January 2008, Issue 80.

Groopman, Jerome. "Epilogue: A Patient's Questions." In *How Doctors Think.* Boston: Houghton Mifflin, 2007.

HealthGrades. "Find a Physician." www.healthgrades.com. (Charges small fee.)

Manning, Phil R., and Lois DeBakey. "Reading: Keeping Current." In *Medicine: Preserving the Passion in the 21st Century,* 2nd ed. New York: Springer, 2003.

National Fibromyalgia Association. "Find a Fibro-Friendly Doctor." www.fmaware.org/site/News2?page=NewsArticle&id=6213.

CHAPTER 4: THE 10 BEST QUESTIONS

To Assess a Doctor After Your First Consultation

> Every human being is the author of his own health or disease.
>
> —Buddha

Seeing a doctor for the first time is like going on a blind date. You want to find someone you can have a trusted relationship with.

Use the 10 Best Questions in this chapter to stop, reflect, and decide how much you liked the new doctor that you've just seen. You are probably going on warp speed at this moment, stressed out by your diagnosis, pain, and fatigue. Your head may feel crammed with a whole new medical language. In other words, you are probably more focused on your disease than your new doctor right now.

Find your favorite quiet spot, draw a soothing bubble bath, or just pull off to the side of the road for a few minutes while you think about your first impressions of the doctor you just met with. You'll have time to review your diagnosis and treatment plan, so this may be one of the few times you can think hard about your new doctor or medical specialist.

If you have your partner or another loved one with you, both of you can discuss the following Best Questions together. It won't take long, and you shouldn't lose this opportunity.

"I am appalled, absolutely appalled, at how little doctors say and how many patients come away not having any idea of their case."
—DR. C. EVERETT KOOP, FORMER U.S. SURGEON GENERAL

>>>THE 10 BEST QUESTIONS
To Assess a Doctor After Your First Consultation

1. How well did the doctor explain my diagnosis in words that I/we could easily understand?

The best doctors don't necessarily use the biggest words. Today, you needed a simple explanation of your diagnosis in plain English, not fancy medical jargon. The best doctors are skillful at explaining complex diseases, medications, and treatment plans in simple terms.

Explaining a new diagnosis, even one as complex as fibromyalgia, is something that most doctors do all the time. Did you understand everything? Did he volunteer facts before you asked for them? Were you offered more information about fibromyalgia and treatment options?

2. How well did the doctor listen to me?

Nonjudgmental listening is the key to the most harmonious and effective doctor-patient relationships. When both parties are listening without bias, they are open to what the other says and thinks. The doctor shouldn't have interrupted you, or derided or belittled anything you said or asked. Having a good listener really matters over the long haul of treating chronic symptoms.

The George Washington University's Dr. Christina M. Puchalski says, "The mark of a good doctor is someone who can treat every patient as an individual and not make hasty conclusions from preconceived notions. A good doctor has to really listen to everything the patient is saying."

3. How well did the doctor react to my questions?

Dr. Jerome Groopman, in his bestselling book *How Doctors Think,* says, "Patients can help the doctor think by asking questions." Another version of this idea is suggested by fibromyalgia expert, Dr. Daniel Clauw, who suggests you ask your doctor, "How can I help you to help me?"

The best doctors react positively to questions instead of becoming annoyed, cynical, or angry. They are open to seeing things from your perspective. If this doctor resented your questions (and you can honestly say that you asked them in a way that was well timed and phrased appropriately), then this negative reaction says more about the doctor than about you and your questions.

There are no dumb questions. You have every right to ask questions. A doctor's lack of essential communication skills can be a deal breaker.

Lynne Matallana explains, "Many people who have fibromyalgia want a doctor who is very compassionate or supportive of their diagnosis of fibromyalgia. Other people prefer a more direct doctor who won't talk down to them and will appreciate the patient's research on his or her condition."

THE QUESTION DOCTOR SAYS:

In addition to reflecting how well this doctor reacted to your questions, also consider how many questions he asked you and how interested he was in your answers. This little insight might say a lot about how likely this doctor is to go the extra mile for you.

4. What did the doctor's body language tell me about his interest and involvement in my care?

Communication experts tell us that most of us unconsciously read body language when we are talking with others. For example, you can probably tell when your children are getting restless, when your partner is grumpy, or when your mother-in-law wants to go home just by the way they sit, stand, or turn their bodies away from you.

The same happens in doctor-patient relationships. The clues may be subtle, but they are powerful. In fact, those same communication experts say that if we get mixed signals, such as if the doctor is saying nice things but looks bored, we unconsciously believe the body language more readily.

5. How comfortable do I feel about working with this doctor?

Comfort level, like trust, is highly subjective. You need a doctor whom you can relax with, who gives off good vibes, and treats you with respect. Your doctor should be interested in you as a person, not just your disease or symptoms, and treat you more like an equal partner in your care rather than a dependent child.

The flip side is not to fall for a doctor with a great bedside manner and personality but nothing between the ears. Asking the Best Questions in this book will help to ensure this doesn't happen.

6. How willing is this doctor to be available after regular office hours?

The best doctors find ways for you to reach them when you need to, especially in the beginning of your treatment process. Doctors in large medical practices or centers typically share their off-hour duty time with partners or have a professional answering service.

Some doctors encourage you to send them e-mails or call their cell phones. How sincere was he in offering you after-hours assistance?

7. Did the doctor spend enough time with me?

This is a tricky one because everyone's perception of "enough time" is different. What matters is how you personally felt about the visit. A good doctor doesn't make you feel rushed—even if you only have a few minutes together—because she gives you her undivided attention.

What you might see as a negative, such as feeling like you were rushed in and out, might be seen as a positive by another patient who has a tight schedule or had to take unpaid time off from work. Notice how long your wait was and how long other patients were waiting. Compare the amount of your wait time with your actual time spent with the doctor.

8. Did this doctor have a problem-solving approach to my treatment plan that included my family?

Your doctor needs good communication skills to deal with your reactions and questions. Likewise, you want your partner, family, or the loved one who accompanied you to this office visit to be treated with respect.

Having a problem-solving approach means that your doctor sees you and your loved ones as part of the team that the doctor is assembling to fight fibromyalgia. The best doctors know how important your support system and loved ones are to your healing.

9. What is my impression of the office staff?

Were you (and your loved ones) greeted warmly? Did the staff seem efficient and courteous? Were your previous medical records or test results ready when you got there? Did they handle your insurance forms well? Were you offered additional assistance?

Or did you feel that you had been dropped into a medical version of a Denny's restaurant, focused on quantity and not the quality of service?

All of these little things add up and can ultimately make a big difference in your overall satisfaction with this doctor. You don't need any more stress in your life.

10. Was this doctor willing to let me tape-record our conversation?

Many of the doctors interviewed for this book believe that it's a good idea for patients to tape-record their sessions with their doctor, even if a loved one also takes notes for you. Some doctors think that taping may protect them legally as well as help their patients be better informed.

This is especially true when you and your doctor are first reviewing your diagnosis, symptoms, important test results, a major procedure, or a change in medications and overall treatment. You can review the tape later and there's less pressure on your accompanying loved one, who may also be nervous, to write rather than listen.

❯ The Magic Question

How much did this doctor try to educate me about my disease?

Charles Mayo, cofounder of the legendary Mayo Clinic, once said, "The safest thing for a patient is to be in the hands of a man engaged in teaching medicine." You want your doctor to be your teacher, willing to explain the rationale behind his recommendations, and equally willing to listen to your opinions and needs.

Reflect back on how much time this doctor spent explaining—teaching you—about your disease and treatment options. It's a wonderful indicator of this doctor's most fundamental belief about a patient as a special person and as a partner—and not just one more patient on a long day's roster.

IN SEARCH OF A DOCTOR I CAN TRUST

It's very important that you have a doctor you trust to help you manage your fibromyalgia effectively. If you dislike your doctor, you are less likely to follow his advice and go for regular check-ups.

Dr. Kim Allan Williams, a senior Chicago-based cardiologist and the current chairperson of the board for the Association of Black Cardiologists, comments, "There's a fair amount of fear for some African-Americans in their relationships with their physicians that often is not expressed."

Likewise, Dr. Rebecca Allison, a Phoenix cardiologist and the 2009 president of the Gay and Lesbian Medical Association, says, "The main concern for a lot of gay, lesbian, bisexual, and transgender patients is being able to confide in their doctors. Many of us are fearful that our doctors will not be very receptive to us."

University of Pennsylvania sleep expert Dr. Charles R. Cantor gives an example why this patient-physician communication is important. He says, "You should feel totally relaxed about discussing your sleep. Some people might be reluctant to discuss the unusual things they are experiencing at night, but they should be forthcoming about it."

If these concerns sound familiar or you want a different doctor for other reasons, use these Best Questions plus the questions in chapters 2 and 3 as your guide. You deserve the best.

CONCLUSION

It's worth it to take the time to assess upfront whether or not you think you have the right doctor for you, especially if you've just recently been diagnosed with fibromyalgia or a related condition. The ideal doctor balances competence with compassion, explaining with listening, and your Best Questions with his "Best Answers."

THE 10 BEST RESOURCES

Groopman, Jerome. "The Eye of the Beholder." In *How Doctors Think*. New York: Houghton Mifflin, 2007.

LeMaitre, George D. *How to Choose A Good Doctor*. Bloomington, IN: AuthorHouse, 2005.

Manning, Phil R., and Lois DeBakey. "Learning by Teaching." *In Medicine: Preserving the Passion in the 21st Century,* 2nd ed. Warren, MI: Springer, 2003.

MedicineNet. "How to Choose a Doctor." www.medicinenet.com/script/main/art.asp?articlekey=47649.

National Fibromyalgia Association. "Achieving a Doctor-Patient Partnership." www.fmaware.org/site/News2?page=NewsArticle&id=6215.

National Fibromyalgia Association. "Good vs. Bad Doctors: How to Tell a Knight on a White Horse from a Jerk on a High Horse." www.fmaware.org/site/News2?page=NewsArticle&id=6217.

Parker-Pope, Tara. "How to Get Treated Like a Doctor Without Going to Medical School." *Wall Street Journal*. February 3, 2004, D1.

Real Simple. "Questions to Ask Your New Doctor." www.realsimple.com/realsimple/content/0,21770,1532440,00.html.

Shomon, Mary J. "Finding and Working with the Best Practitioners." In *Living Well with Chronic Fatigue Syndrome and Fibromyalgia: What*

Your Doctor Doesn't Tell You . . . That You Need to Know. New York: HarperCollins, 2004.

U.S. Department of Health & Human Services, Agency for Healthcare Research and Quality. "Build Your Question List." www.ahrq.gov/questionsaretheanswer/questionBuilder.aspx.

CHAPTER 5: THE 10 BEST QUESTIONS

To Ask When Getting a Second Opinion

One doctor makes work for another.

—English proverb

Seriously consider getting a second opinion about your diagnosis of fibromyalgia. This disease is still misunderstood and misdiagnosed by much of the medical community. If you are seeing a primary care physician who has limited experience with fibromyalgia, consider getting a second opinion from a top "fibro-friendly" specialist or medical treatment center. See chapters 2, 3, and 4.

Getting an accurate diagnosis from a medical expert who is knowledgeable in fibromyalgia can help you greatly. He will recognize your symptoms, clarify if you have fibromyalgia or a related disorder, and get you started on an effective treatment plan. You may also want a second opinion about your prescription medications or almost any aspect of your medical care, including a specialist's help with specific symptoms. For example, you may benefit from a second opinion and a sleep study from a sleep expert. Another common reason for second opinions is to find another doctor because you dislike or distrust your current one.

Second opinions are becoming increasingly common due to two current trends. First, patients are becoming more involved, empowered, and knowledgeable about their own medical care. Secondly, with the rapidly growing medical interest in fibromyalgia, there are more treatment options than ever before.

Don't worry about offending your current doctor or challenging his expertise. The best doctors welcome second opinions and even seek out additional advice for themselves. If your current doctor strongly objects, his reaction may be a red flag warning that he lacks experience or self-confidence for treating fibromyalgia or related symptoms.

Remember, it's your health and well-being that's ultimately at stake here. Dr. Vicki Rackner, a Washington-based patient advocate and author, is a strong believer in the value of second opinions. She says simply, "You need a second opinion for everything."

On balance, before you seek a second opinion double-check your own motives. You may be the product of a long, ugly crusade to get a correct diagnosis and still harbor resentment about how you've been treated. Sometimes people with fibromyalgia who are bitter or angry take out their frustrations on their new doctors, even the supportive ones.

Fibromyalgia expert Dr. Michael McNett further explains, "Skepticism and even scorn are far too common in the medical profession concerning fibromyalgia. But it's very important that patients *not* carry their negative feelings or experiences into a new doctor's office. If the patient comes in with a chip on her shoulder, she will dramatically increase the likelihood that they will have an unproductive interaction."

Check with your insurance plan or Medicare to see if it will pay for a second opinion. Don't feel rushed about finding and consulting a second-opinion doctor. A delay usually won't impact your prognosis. Make sure you verify this with your doctor.

This chapter's Best Questions are a little different. Ask *yourself* the first five Best Questions to help you decide if you really want a second opinion, especially if you must pay for it yourself. Ask the *second-opinion doctor* questions 6 through 10 when you are meeting with her to discuss your case.

>>>THE 10 BEST QUESTIONS
To Ask When Getting a Second Opinion

Best Questions to Ask Yourself *Before Seeking a Second Opinion*

1. How do I rate my current doctor's knowledge about my disease and her ability to support me well during treatment?

Many patients underestimate what they should know about fibromyalgia and its treatment. Other patients, who sometimes spend years trying to get an accurate diagnosis, know more about fibromyalgia than their doctors.

Medical specialists, such as rheumatologists, will be more knowledgeable about fibromyalgia than most primary care physicians or internists. You want a doctor you can count on, especially since fibromyalgia is a chronic disease and impacts your quality of life.

2. How confident am I in my current doctor's interest in treating me as a unique person?

You're trying to assess if your current doctor is a great, good, or just a mediocre doctor. Think back to your doctor's treatment plan for you. How comprehensive was it? Did she seem sincerely interested in you as an individual? Did she fully explain your treatment options? Do you feel you can trust her?

By all means, avoid highly opinionated doctors who prescribe the same drugs or treatment plans over and over again for almost all of their patients. Legendary psychologist Abraham Maslow once noted that when all you have is a hammer, everything looks like a nail. The same applies here. When a doctor only knows a small handful of treatment options, every patient looks the same—like a nail in pain.

3. How much do I understand about what I've been told to date about my diagnosis and treatment options?

Reflect on your prior discussions with your doctor. Look over your notes. Scan this book to learn more about treatment options. All of this will help the factual information to sink in as you step back to assess your situation for a moment.

Now with this cleared head, think through how much you truly understand. This is not a reflection on your intelligence but rather a sign of how well your current doctor has explained your diagnosis and treatment plan.

You want a doctor who is willing and capable of putting medical jargon into easy-to-understand terms. The word *doctor* is from the Latin *docere,* meaning "to teach." The medical profession has evolved over time, and now we think of doctoring and teaching as two separate functions. But look for a good doctor who is also willing to be your teacher and partner.

4. How complicated are my symptoms and treatment plan?

If you think you have a straightforward fibromyalgia case, don't assume there are no pending decisions or you don't need to educate yourself. In most cases you still have choices, such as how aggressively you want to be treated with prescription medications versus alternative therapies.

The doctor's beliefs, customs, financial practices, medical education, and available resources are factors behind the scenes that influence her decisions and are usually not obvious to patients. Your doctor's recommendations are based on her subjective assessment of your case. Doctors are only human and can make mistakes.

5. What does my inner voice tell me is right for me?

There's a lot to be said for the value of going with your gut-level reaction. After you've asked all the highly logical, rational, analytical questions, you should also listen to your inner voice.

Malcolm Gladwell, the author of *Blink,* would agree. He says, "We really only trust conscious decision making. But there are moments, particularly in times of stress, when haste does not make waste, when our snap judgments and first impressions can offer a much better means of making sense of the world. . . . Decisions made very quickly can be every bit as good as decisions made cautiously and deliberately."

THE QUESTION DOCTOR SAYS:

Use questions 6 through 10 to ask a second-opinion doctor about your diagnosis and treatment, or just to find a doctor you'll like better. Before you begin your doctor search, get a clear idea of what kind of doctor you want and why.

Best Questions to Ask the Doctor *When Getting a Second Opinion*

6. How do you interpret my symptoms?

Ask the second doctor to perform the tender point exam or review the previous doctor's fibromyalgia diagnosis. Medical experts and patients disagree about whether your second opinion should be "blind." A blind second opinion means that the first doctor's opinion and sometimes the original diagnosis aren't shared with the second doctor.

The advantage is that the blind second opinion will be more

objective and not influenced by the first one. The drawbacks include putting your second-opinion doctor at a disadvantage by not letting him know about the original diagnosis. Another option is to provide information about your symptoms without including the first doctor's diagnosis or treatment recommendations.

7. What are the chances that my diagnosis is incorrect?

Fibromyalgia symptoms may not be recognized by a doctor who sees few cases or is inexperienced in using the tender point diagnostic exam. Men with fibromyalgia are less likely to be diagnosed correctly because many doctors assume it's a "women's disease." In addition, many overlapping conditions, such as sleep apnea (breathing difficulties during sleep), or other medical conditions, such as diabetes or heart disease, may be overlooked or misdiagnosed as the doctor focuses solely on treating your pain and fatigue.

8. In your opinion, have my symptoms been properly diagnosed and described? Please explain the rationale for your answer.

This is a straightforward question that goes to the heart of why you want a second opinion. Make sure the second doctor takes the time to fully explain her reasoning behind her assessment of your case. Don't hesitate to ask any other questions about specific symptoms to understand what you're being told.

9. Are there any alternative forms of treatment available that my previous doctor may have overlooked? What treatments do you recommend for me?

Not all doctors are equally supportive of alternative therapies, such as healthy diet and exercise choices, acupuncture, and dietary supplements. But there is growing evidence-based research within the context of rigorous science that some complementary and alternative therapies (also called **integrative medicine**) have value.

The federal government's National Center for Complementary and Alternative Medicine has an informative Web site (http://nccam.nih.gov). See chapters 9 and 10 on alternative therapies. A second opinion that includes a look at alternative therapies may expand your treatment options in ways that your primary care physician hadn't previously considered.

10. In your opinion, what is my prognosis after going through the treatment plan you've outlined?

Try to refrain from asking this question too early in the discussion. This way you can really listen to everything else the doctor has to say and make a well-informed decision about whether you like his treatment plan, personal style, and potential to support you in the upcoming months. Pay attention to how detailed and personalized his answer is to this question.

THE QUESTION DOCTOR SAYS:

Reduce the cost and time required for a second opinion by asking your first doctor to send copies of all tests results to the second-opinion doctor if you choose not to have a blind second opinion. Take a friend or family member, a notepad, and a tape recorder to this office visit. That way you'll be able to listen and can compare later notes and recordings between the first and second doctors.

❯ The Magic Question

What advice would you give to your mother (sister, wife) to help her choose between the different recommendations/diagnoses/treatment options I've received?

If the first and second doctors disagree on your diagnosis or treatment plan, you may be confronted with a situation in which you have to choose between them without really knowing which one is better.

Rather than trying to be the Lone Ranger here and solve this problem yourself, this Magic Question will put the second-opinion doctor's thinking cap on and engage him in helping you make the best decision. If needed, you can also go back to your first doctor and ask this same question and then compare answers.

Another strategy is to ask the two doctors to confer on your case and see if they can arrive at a mutual decision. You might also want to ask for a third opinion and then compare.

CONCLUSION

Why get a second opinion? The fundamental question when you are considering second opinions is really, "Why not?"

Asking for a second opinion is a frequent practice, growing more common, and some insurance companies even recommend or require it. Don't worry about insulting a doctor's intelligence, even if he's your old favorite family doctor. The best doctors will actively support you.

THE 10 BEST RESOURCES

About.com. Adrienne Dellwo's Fibromyalgia & Chronic Fatigue Blog. "Do You Need a Second Opinion?" http://chronicfatigue.about .com/b/2007/08/11/do-you-need-a-second-opinion.htm.

About.com "When Do You Need a Second Opinion?" http://patients .about.com/od/discoveringyourdiagnosis/a/need2nd opinion.htm.

Centers for Medicare & Medicaid Services. "Getting a Second Opinion Before Surgery." www.medicare.gov/Publications/Pubs/pdf/02173.pdf.

Gladwell, Malcolm. *Blink: The Power of Thinking Without Thinking.* New York: Little, Brown, 2005.

Groopman, Jerome. "The Uncertainty of the Expert." In *How Doctors Think.* Boston: Houghton Mifflin, 2007.

Gruman, Jessie. AfterShock: *What to Do When the Doctor Gives You—Or Someone You Love—a Devastating Diagnosis.* New York: Walker & Company, 2007.

Levine, Evan. *What Your Doctor Won't (or Can't) Tell You: The Failures of American Medicine—and How to Avoid Becoming a Statistic.* New York: Berkley Trade, 2005.

National Fibromyalgia Association. "How Can I Help My Child with Fibromyalgia?"www.fmaware.org/site/News2?page=NewsArticle&id=6044.

U.S. Department of Health & Human Services. Agency for Healthcare Research and Quality. "Quick Tips—When Talking with Your Doctor." www.ahrq.gov/consumer/quicktips/doctalk.htm.

Wrongdiagnosis.com. "How Common Is Misdiagnosis?" www.wrong diagnosis.com/intro/common.htm.

CHAPTER 6: THE 10 BEST QUESTIONS
For Wellness Checkups

The only way to keep your health is to eat what you don't want, drink what you don't like, and do what you'd druther not.

—Mark Twain

After you've been diagnosed with fibromyalgia, it's very important to continue getting routine wellness checkups with your primary care physician or internist. A wellness checkup prevents or tracks other ongoing illnesses you may have, such as heart disease or diabetes. It also considers your risk factors for developing certain diseases later in life.

Dr. Patrick Wood, a Seattle-based fibromyalgia expert comments, "Some physicians attribute essentially everything to fibromyalgia and may overlook treatment, assuming that because it's fibromyalgia, it's not treatable. This is absurd. People with fibromyalgia get sick, too."

During the exam your doctor will check your weight, blood pressure, and other vital signs. He will request standard blood tests, such as a complete blood count (CBC) and a urine analysis.

This chapter focuses on non-fibromyalgia health concerns. Use the following Best Questions as a guide to your conversation with your doctor during your wellness checkup and when discussing test results. Asking these questions will keep you more actively involved in your own health and well-being. Be sure to also ask specific questions about your own health concerns, symptoms, or conditions other than fibromyalgia.

THE QUESTION DOCTORS SAYS:

Consider focusing on just one or two risk factors or Best Questions if you want a more in-depth discussion with your doctor. You might make better use of your time together by just discussing your weight, family medical history, or smoking, for example.

>>>THE 10 BEST QUESTIONS
For Wellness Checkups

1. What is my ideal weight? How can I achieve it? What is my BMI? What is my hip-to-waist measurement?

That Americans' waistlines have expanded is a well known fact. Obesity has doubled since the 1970s, and now at least 62 percent of adults in the United States are overweight or obese. The official definition of obese is being thirty or more pounds overweight.

The more you weigh, the more likely you are to have a heart attack earlier in life. To properly assess your weight-related heart risks, you need three numbers: 1) your weight in pounds, 2) your body mass index (BMI), which is a key measure of obesity, and 3) your hip-to-waist ratio.

Ask your doctor for a body mass index (BMI) test, a simple, quick test of your body's fatness. An ideal BMI is 25 or less, and a BMI over 30 is considered obese.

A 2008 Duke University study found a significant link was found between BMI, obesity, and heart attack risk. The average age for a first heart attack for those with a BMI over forty was only 58.7 years. Women's heart disease risks increase significantly with age, especially after menopause.

Ask your doctor to measure your waist-to-hip ratio, which is related to your body shape. People with excessive weight around the waist (so-called apple shape) are at greater risk than people who are heavier below the waist (pear shape). A waist-to-hip ratio of more than 0.9 (or forty inches) for men or 0.85 (or thirty-five inches) for women indicates an increase in heart risks. New studies in the *Journal of the American College of Cardiology* found that the waist-to-hip ratio predicts cardiovascular risks better than BMI.

Judge your own weight, BMI, and hip-to-waist ratio using the Centers for Disease Control and Prevention's Web site at www .cdc.gov/nccdphp/dnpa/healthyweight/assessing/index.htm. Losing weight isn't easy. Ask your doctor for specific advice. Chapter 16 has more diet tips.

2. What foods should I eat? What type of diet do you recommend for me?

Currently, the most commonly recommended diet is the Mediterranean diet filled with fruits, vegetables, fiber, grains, healthy fish, and olive oils.

One smart question that you might not think to ask your doctor is, "How can I take my favorite foods and make them healthier?" For example, Dr. Kim Allan Williams, the current chairman of the Association of Black Cardiologists, suggests, "Take soul food, reduce the salt, and replace the meat with a soy product, such as soy sausages, chicken, or burgers. Use olive oil instead of lard. If you replace the meat, sodium, and lard, you're doing pretty well."

3. What are my cholesterol numbers for HDL, LDL, and triglycerides? What do my cholesterol numbers indicate about my heart risks? How can I improve my cholesterol?

Knowing your HDL, LDL, and triglyceride levels is important wellness information. These are the three blood particles that make up your total **lipid count** or the fatty substances in your blood collectively called **cholesterol.** Cutting-edge research indicates that you should *not* focus on your total cholesterol number but rather know all three HDL, LDL, and triglyceride numbers.

With **HDL (good) cholesterol,** higher levels are better. Heart risks happen with low HDL levels (lower than 40 mg/dL for men, lower than 50 mg/dL for women). Normal levels range from 40 to 60 mg/dL. Above 60 mg/dL is considered heart protective.

The lower your **LDL (bad) cholesterol,** the lower your risk of heart disease. LDL cholesterol is the bad fat in your arteries. Lower than 100 mg/dL is optimal, and a level of 190 mg/dL and above is a very high risk. (Associate H with high and L with low to remember the difference between the "good" and "bad" cholesterols.)

Triglycerides are a type of fat. The normal level is lower than 150 mg/dL, borderline high is 150–199 mg/dL, and too high is 200 mg/dL and up.

A toxic combination is low HDL (good) and high triglyceride levels. This is called **metabolic syndrome.** People with metabolic syndrome have the highest risk for developing heart disease and diabetes. See more at www.americanheart.org/presenter .jhtml?identifier=4756.

Don't settle for just your total cholesterol number from your doctor. Ask her to explain the details of your profile. Blood cholesterol is complicated. For example, there are seven types of LDL (bad) cholesterol and five types of HDL (good) cholesterol.

In addition, many researchers now think that blood cholesterol is *not* the best predictor of heart disease risk. Some people who have a heart attack don't have high cholesterol levels.

Dr. H. Robert Superko, an executive director at St. Joseph's Translational Research Institute in Atlanta, explains, "Cholesterol is a major cause of heart disease in people who have high cholesterol, but most people don't have high cholesterol. What the drug companies want you to believe is that if you just take our drug (statins) you'll be fine. But the truth is that a 25 percent relative heart attack risk reduction is not good enough. This 25 percent reduction means that if 100 people NOT taking the drug have a heart attack, 75 people taking the drug still have a heart attack."

The bottom line is you want to cut your risks by reducing the bad (LDL) cholesterol in your blood, eat healthier, get regular exercise, and, if needed, take cholesterol reducing drugs, such as **statins** or **bile binding resins**.

4. What is my blood pressure? What can I do to better manage my blood pressure?

High blood pressure (also called **hypertension**) is defined as a systolic pressure (top number) of 140 mm Hg or higher and/or a diastolic pressure (bottom number) of 90 mm Hg or higher. The ideal number combination is lower than 120 (systolic, top) over lower than 80 (diastolic, bottom).

Hypertension is often underdiagnosed and under-treated. It is a "silent killer" that affects about 65 million Americans and 1 billion people worldwide. High blood pressure directly increases your risk of heart and other diseases. It is especially prevalent among African-Americans and people who are elderly, obese, heavy drinkers, and diabetics.

Dr. Kim Allan Williams advises, "African-Americans have more complications from high blood pressure (hypertension)." Statistically, African-Americans have one of the highest hypertension rates in the world (35 percent).

Know your numbers by having your blood pressure checked often. Eat fewer processed foods and lose your salt shaker.

Good follow-up questions to ask your doctor include:

- How often should I check my blood pressure?
- Should I buy a home blood pressure monitor?
- Do I need to take blood pressure medicine?
- What's my ideal daily salt (sodium) limit?

5. What is my risk of developing diabetes? Or, how can I best manage my diabetes?

Diabetes is deadly. It occurs when the body doesn't produce or properly use insulin, the hormone needed to convert sugar and starches into body energy. The American Diabetes Association states that 23.6 million Americans (7.8 percent) have diabetes. Nearly 6 million people are unaware they have the disease.

Doctors test for diabetes or prediabetes with either the fasting plasma glucose test (FPG) or the oral glucose tolerance test (OGTT). The American Diabetes Association recommends the FPG because it is easier, faster, and less expensive.

Type 2 diabetes is the most common form. This is a serious but manageable disease. If you are told you have diabetes, prediabetes, or glucose intolerance, be sure you understand your increased risks and what actions you need to take, including prescription drugs and lifestyle adjustments. Two large research studies concluded you *can* prevent or manage Type 2 diabetes with a healthy diet and regular exercise.

6. What physical activity (exercise) do you recommend for me now and later?

Chances are you need more physical activity, but you find it challenging due to your fibromyalgia. Ask your doctor for practical suggestions about gentle yet consistent exercise routines that you'll enjoy.

Think of exercise as play instead of work. Exercise doesn't have to be strenuous or boring. Bill Sonnemaker, MS, an award-winning personal trainer in Atlanta, suggests, "The activity you choose needs to be specific to the improvements you want from your body."

Ask your doctor these additional follow-up questions:

- How much exercise and what types of exercise do you recommend for me?
- What is my target heart rate during exercise? (number of heartbeats per minute)
- What are my exercise limitations and precautions?

7. What can I do to quit smoking or drinking too much alcohol?

Ask your doctor for help, advice, and medications if your smoking or drinking habits are difficult to break. Some people with fibromyalgia find that their increased stress levels or depression contribute to their continued use of tobacco or alcohol even though they want to quit.

The American Lung Association's tobacco control manager Bill Blatt advises, "The biggest obstacle for many smokers is they think it's just a willpower thing. Smoking is not just a bad habit. It's an addiction." Dr. Edwin B. Fisher, a smoking behavior expert at the University of North Carolina, adds, "The real issue is that the more people can personalize the reasons they want to quit, the more they will be able to stay off cigarettes."

If you are concerned about your alcohol consumption habits, alcohol expert Dr. David J. Hanson, a professor emeritus at the State University of New York, suggests you ask yourself, "Has my drinking caused me any problems?"

Good follow-up questions to ask your doctor are, "How can I manage my stress levels or depression while I'm quitting tobacco or alcohol?" and "Do you recommend prescription medications (like nicotine replacement drugs) to help me?"

8. What are my genetic risk factors and what can I do about them?

Some genetic risk factors are well documented, such as heart disease and cancer, while other genetic links are barely understood. You are wise to stay on top of the newest research and ask for less-common tests if you have any suspected genetic predispositions. Regardless of your genetic risks, living a healthy lifestyle will help you.

An important follow-up question is to ask your doctor if you need to tell your children about their possibility of having an inherited disease. For example, Stanford University's Kathy Berra explains, "It's a family affair. Your heart risk factors can be passed on to your son's and daughter's hearts, too."

9. What am I doing *right* that I should keep on doing or do more of?

Okay, the odds are that even if you love deep-fried Oreos, there's something about your health, diet, or weight that you've actually done right up until now. Hearing a small piece of good news boosts your morale.

There's no sense in stopping your good habits while trying to fix your bad habits. For example, your daily glass of wine or beer may be protecting your heart more than you realize, according to a 2008 Harvard study that found moderate drinking was associated with a lower risk of heart attack.

10. How often should I see you for checkups? How can I communicate with you or your office in between appointments if I have questions or concerns?

Be sure to ask these important questions at the end of your office visit, especially if you have other chronic ailments in addition to fibromyalgia. Don't leave the doctor's office second-guessing his answers.

❯ The Magic Question

What are my other, less obvious risk factors?

There are numerous intertwined risk factors linked to a wide diversity of diseases that researchers are only starting to understand.

For example, a 2008 article in the journal *Circulation* called on experts to study a possible connection between sleep apnea (breathing irregularities during sleep) and cardiovascular disease. In a 2007 study, *JAMA* (*The Journal of the American Medical Association*) reported connections between heart disease and bowel cancer. People typically ignore leg pain as a warning sign of blood clots.

Many doctors won't think to consider your additional "hidden" risk factors, so take the initiative by asking this important question.

CONCLUSION

Even if you are seeing your primary care physician for fibromyalgia treatment, don't let your regular wellness checkups slide.

You CAN control your disease and health by living a healthier lifestyle. Family history is not destiny. Cleveland Clinic's preventive medicine consultant Dr. Caldwell B. Esselstyn concludes, "Your genes 'load the gun,' but your lifestyle 'pulls the trigger.'"

THE 10 BEST RESOURCES

American Heart Association. "Heart Attack/Coronary Heart Disease Risk Assessment." www.americanheart.org/presenter.jhtml?identifier=3003499.

CalorieControl.org. "Weight Maintenance Calculator." www.calorie control.org/calcalcs.html.

FamilyDoctor.org. "Tips for Talking with Your Doctor." http://familydoctor
.org/online/famdocen/home/pat-advocacy/healthcare/837.html.

Healthfinder.gov. www.healthfinder.gov. (Provides links for 1,500 organizations and publications.)

Matallana, Lynne, and Laurence A. Bradley, Stuart Silverman, and Muhammad B. Yunus. "Healthy Lifestyle Changes: Exercise and Diet." In *The Complete Idiot's Guide to Fibromyalgia*. New York: Penguin, 2005.

MedicineNet. "Home." www.medicinenet.com/script/main/hp.asp.

MedlinePlus. "Home." http://medlineplus.gov.

National Cholesterol Education Program. "Risk Assessment Tool for Estimating Your 10-Year Risk of Having a Heart Attack." http://hp2010
.nhlbihin.net/atpiii/calculator.asp?usertype=pub.

National Institutes of Health. "PubMed Central." Portal to a free digital archive of medical journals. www.pubmedcentral.nih.gov.

WebMD. "Home." www.webmd.com.

CHAPTER 7: THE 10 BEST QUESTIONS
For Men with Fibromyalgia

A man too busy to take care of his health is like a
mechanic too busy to take care of his tools.

—Spanish proverb

Some people are surprised to learn that fibromyalgia is a guy
thing, too. Fibromyalgia occurs seven times more frequently
in women than men according to the American College of
Rheumatology. Other sources state that 90 percent of fibromyalgia
cases are women, compared to 10 percent men, of the estimated
3 to 6 million Americans with this disease. Still other sources say
that men constitute 25 to 30 percent of all fibromyalgia cases. No
one really knows for sure.

Whatever the numbers, that's still a whole lot of guys in a
whole lot of pain.

Considering how difficult it is for many women to get their fibromyalgia diagnosed correctly, most men have an even tougher
time. Few doctors understand fibromyalgia in men and tend to attribute a man's symptoms to dozens of other causes before considering "that woman's disease, fibromyalgia."

Another problem is highlighted by fibromyalgia expert, Dr.
Kim Dupree Jones. She says, "Men are underrepresented in fibromyalgia in part because of the tender point test. Since men are
more muscular, we probably need to press a little harder during
the initial diagnosis. When doctors start to use more pressure to
diagnose men, I think we are going to see numbers more like 70
percent women, 30 men, not the current 90–10 ratio."

For guys, it's hard enough having a disease like fibromyalgia that few people understand or sympathize with. After all, you don't look sick. But even worse are the myths and misunderstandings about fibromyalgia that may delay your pain management and symptom relief.

Most men with fibromyalgia struggle with constant pain on a daily basis. Their additional burden is dealing with the stigma in our society that real men don't cry. Real men are supposed to just suck it up and soldier through pain like the prizefighter Rocky.

There is a growing consensus among specialists that fibromyalgia does affect men and women differently, but those differences are only beginning to be understood. An example is the gender differences in how the brain's serotonin system (linked to pain, sleep, and depression) functions. Ask your doctor the following Best Questions to ensure you are getting the very best health care possible.

THE QUESTION DOCTOR SAYS:

Take charge of your disease by learning everything you can about it. You need answers. Choose a doctor who welcomes your questions and understands that fibromyalgia in men really does happen.

>>>THE 10 BEST QUESTIONS
For Men with Fibromyalgia

1. Have I gotten all the appropriate tests, procedures, and treatments I need? Are there any other tests, procedures, or treatments that I need now or later?

The odds are that as a man you are less likely to receive the full range of tests, procedures, medications, or alternative options that women with fibromyalgia routinely receive. Nearly every fibromyalgia patient has heard, "It's all in your head." But men are widely underdiagnosed.

Your symptoms may be even more discounted by doctors who don't acknowledge fibromyalgia's existence, much less in men. Even worse, some unenlightened doctors view men with fibromyalgia suspiciously either as drug addicts wanting another pain killer fix, depressive personalities, or exercise flunkouts.

It will be hard to know if you are getting a good answer from your doctor because diagnoses and treatment options vary so widely. A best response is your doctor's thoughtful reconsideration of your medical records rather than a snap answer, "Of course." Make him think twice about *your* case so you don't get just routine cookie-cutter care or the brush-off.

2. Have these tests or drugs that you are recommending been validated for men? Have my previous test results been interpreted accurately based on my gender?

There are many tests or drugs your doctor may recommend for you to the point that you think you've taken every test or drug under the sun.

It's appropriate to ask if a recommended test or drug has been proved effective for men in clinical trials. Researchers still know so little about fibromyalgia, especially in men, that you may not be getting the right tests to exclude other possible diagnoses or the correct drug dosages.

Ask, "Have gender studies been done on this test or drug? What were the results?" Many prescribed medications used for fibromyalgia haven't been as thoroughly researched for men as for women.

A "no" response doesn't automatically mean you shouldn't take a certain drug. Again, this question should prompt your doctor to think more carefully about your care.

3. Could my fibromyalgia/symptoms be caused by a genetic link?

If you have a mother or sister who has been diagnosed with fibromyalgia, you may be able to get a more accurate diagnosis because the doctor is more likely to believe your own symptoms. You may also have an important clue into why you have fibromyalgia in the first place.

In addition, if you share information with your doctor about your family's history of fibromyalgia, you may be ahead of the game in planning your own care. Don't discount a possible genetic link until researchers know with more certainty what causes fibromyalgia. The current thinking is that there is some kind of family connection.

4. Could my fibromyalgia have been caused by my Gulf War (or other war) service?

No one knows exactly what causes fibromyalgia, but if you are a Gulf War veteran or the veteran of another war your condition may be linked to your war service. As fibromyalgia expert Dr. Michael McNett explains, "Trauma and stress can contribute to getting this disease, but they are not considered primary causes." Other doctors believe trauma (both physical and emotional) is a leading cause of fibromyalgia.

If you returned from a war with the symptoms of fibromyalgia, check with the Department of Veterans Affairs (VA) about qualifying for benefits and compensation (www.va.gov). There may be deadlines on your eligibility, so check sooner rather than later with the VA.

5. What are your recommendations for my overall treatment plan?

Your overall treatment plan should be a good balance between over-the-counter medications and prescription drugs, along with suggestions for lifestyle changes and alternative therapies. Make sure the doctor talks about short-term and long-term treatment strategies.

See other chapters and the resource list at the end of this book for more information on treatments.

6. What diet, exercise, and other lifestyle changes do you suggest for me?

Your doctor should address her answer to this question from the perspective of your unique case, medical history, and the fact that you are a man with fibromyalgia. Ask questions about any suggestions that don't sound realistic or doable.

Part III of this book has more specific questions, if needed. There are also many Web sites and other books available on adopting a healthy lifestyle when living with fibromyalgia.

7. Where can I get more factual and medical information on fibromyalgia in men?

Your doctor will probably refer you to the National Fibromyalgia Association (www.fmaware.org) for good general information and perhaps PubMed Central for medical information (www.ncbi.nlm .nih.gov/sites/entrez?db=PubMed). Be sure to do your own Internet searches to find more that is useful to you, but be wary of Web sites selling "cures." Chapter 10 explains why.

8. Where can I get emotional and personal support?

Chances are if you are a man with fibromyalgia you are angry about it—or have been. You may have spent years trying to get a correct diagnosis, continually criticized by doctors and family alike about your "imagined" complaints, or seen an important relationship dissolve, all due to fibromyalgia. You may even have been criticized for not being "a manly man."

Dr. Michael McNett observes, "The disease is fairly similar in both men and women, but what's different is the social stigma for men. For example, in our society, it's socially acceptable for men to get angry but not sad or depressed."

Fibromyalgia isn't sexy or fun. It can rock a guy's self-image as he goes from being the family breadwinner or a great basketball player to being increasingly disabled and dependent. One day you can shoot hoops, and the next day you can barely get out of bed.

Asking for emotional help isn't sissy; it's smart. If your doctor doesn't know or you don't want to join a women-only fibromyalgia support group, try some of the online chat rooms for men listed in the resources below.

9. How are my sexual performance and sexual pleasure likely to be affected by my fibromyalgia and prescribed medications?

There are some medications that are commonly prescribed for fibromyalgia or related symptoms that may affect your sexual performance and pleasure. In addition, you may find certain sexual positions uncomfortable or impossible due to pain or fatigue.

Because of the emphasis many men and couples put on sexual capabilities, these changes may be very distressing for you. Having an honest conversation with your doctor may go a long way to boosting your self-confidence in the bedroom. Another way to ask this question is, "Does my having fibromyalgia have any implications for my masculinity?" Also see chapter 21 on sex and intimacy.

10. What symptoms are serious enough that I should call you? How can I best reach you?

Rather than second-guessing when to call your doctor or being reluctant to because you don't want to bother him, get the straight facts now based on your personal medical history.

Some doctors will gladly give you their cell phone numbers or e-mail addresses, and others won't. Find out your doctor's preferred communication mode and availability before you have to guess.

❯ The Magic Question

What's the latest thing you read or learned about men and fibromyalgia?

This is a repeated Magic Question from chapter 3, this time with a "man's" angle. As a man with fibromyalgia, it's absolutely vital that you have a doctor who knows (and cares about) the latest research on how this disease affects men differently from women.

CONCLUSION

If you are a man with fibromyalgia, you are not alone and you are not nuts. Lynne Matallana, president of the National Fibromyalgia Association, advises, "What's important for men is to go to a doctor who understands that fibromyalgia does not discriminate between men and women. Good doctors recognize that men may have different issues or questions that they are dealing with. For example, men are not allowed to have pain or admit that they have it in our society."

This is not the time to be passive or pissed off. Consider your diagnosis of fibromyalgia as your wakeup call to look out for Number One and take better care of yourself.

Be proactive. Ask these Best Questions and any other questions important to you. Stick to your guns and learn as much as you can about your disease, your own case, and especially about the factors that you can control with a healthy lifestyle.

THE 10 BEST RESOURCES

ClinicalTrials.gov. "Fibromyalgia in Men Suffering from PTSD." www.clinicaltrials.gov/ct2/show/NCT00229294?term=fibromyalgia&rank-118.

Fibromyalgia-Symptoms.org. "Men with Fibromyalgia." www.fibromyalgia-symptoms.org/fibromyalgia_relieve.html.

The Institute for Molecular Medicine. "Gulf War Illnesses Research." www.immed.org/illness/gulfwar_illness_research.html.

Medscape Today. "Trauma as Precipitating Event for Fibromyalgia Syndrome." http://www.medscape.com/viewarticle/470556_5.

Men with Fibromyalgia. "Forums." www.menwithfibro.com/forum/index.php?PHPSESSID=4be79de0d9b6b8dac027bc655dc60ad9.

Men with Fibromyalgia. "Home." www.menwithfibro.com/home.html.

National Fibromyalgia Association. "Men with Fibromyalgia." www.fmaware.org/site/PageServer?pagename=topics_menWithFM.

National Fibromyalgia Association. "The Paradox of Pain: A Male Perspective." www.fmaware.org/site/News2?page=NewsArticle&id=5314.

Neurotransmitter.net. "Fibromyalgia Genetics." www.neurotransmitter.net/fibromyalgiagenetic.html.

Peter's Fibromyalgia & Personal Website. "What Do You Do First?" www.merlinean.com/tinyd4+index.id+1.htm.

PART II:

Choosing Treatments

Being diagnosed with fibromyalgia is often terribly upsetting. Many people are especially devastated to learn that there is no known cause or cure. Other people with fibromyalgia are relieved to know that they aren't crazy and there is actually a disease with a medical name to describe their often baffling symptoms.

Most people with a new diagnosis feel overwhelmed, depressed, or panicked. You may find you are facing important decisions about choosing medications or therapies, but feel confused about knowing all the facts or where to turn for advice.

There are many uniquely personal reactions to fibromyalgia. Not everyone wants to do a lot of research or become a walking encyclopedia on it, yet others wouldn't have it any other way. Some people reach out for alternative therapies for pain relief and to dozens of people for comfort and advice, while others choose conservative treatments and prefer privacy.

The 10 Best Questions in this section will help to strengthen your decision-making muscles. Because fibromyalgia isn't curable, you and your doctor will look for the best ways to minimize your pain and fatigue with a combination of drugs, alternative therapies, and healthy lifestyle changes.

Sorting through your personal priorities and learning about your treatment options will bring you a greater measure of comfort and self-confidence. Chapter 8 suggests what to ask your doctor about fibromyalgia medications. If you want to know more about alternative therapies and how to avoid being ripped off by a scam artist or bogus Web sites, see chapters 9 and 10. Use chapter 12 to find a great massage therapist and chapter 13 to choose a top acupuncturist.

The Question Doctor sincerely hopes the following Best Questions will ease your journey. Being an empowered patient is all about having the knowledge and strength to ask lots of good questions. Here is your script.

About Fibromyalgia Medications

It is easy to get a thousand prescriptions but hard to get one single remedy.

—Chinese proverb

Fibromyalgia medications are a good news–bad news story. The good news is that because there is a growing acceptance within the medical community of fibromyalgia as a "real disease," large pharmaceutical companies are racing to develop fibromyalgia medications (and make profits). Fibromyalgia expert Dr. Michael McNett comments, "Now that several drugs are in the pipeline and several have been approved, 'big pharm's' muscle is coming to bear and it's helping to teach doctors about fibromyalgia."

Oregon fibromyalgia expert Dr. Kim Dupree Jones agrees, "Science has made enough progress on what's wrong biologically in fibromyalgia that we can now use the right drugs to target specific problems and not just mask symptoms."

The bad news is that there is no magic bullet in a bottle for fibromyalgia. Linda Pütz, a career coach with fibromyalgia reflects on her difficulties, "I began my journey of experimenting with medications and having my hopes dashed over and over again that I would be in less pain and be able to sleep better."

It usually takes experimenting with a combination of medications and dosages to find the best "cocktail" to meet your needs. Dr. Patrick Wood, a fibromyalgia expert in Seattle explains, "People can have complicated drug regimens because there are so many targets to shoot at because there is so much going on." For example, many people with fibromyalgia need medications not only for widespread pain relief but also for symptoms including sleep disorders, depression, irritable bowel syndrome, and painful menstrual cycles.

Ask your doctor the following Best Questions about her recommendations for medications and your general treatment plan. Be sure to check with your insurance provider or Medicare about payment coverage details.

THE QUESTION DOCTOR SAYS:

Consider taking a tape recorder or a notepad with you when you see your doctor. Many people are intimidated by discussions about complex drugs with long, unpronounceable names. You can listen to the tape or review your notes later without the additional pressure of being face to face with the doctor. Ask your doctor to write down both the generic and brand names for any drugs she prescribes for you.

〉〉〉THE 10 BEST QUESTIONS
About Fibromyalgia Medications

1. What drugs do you recommend I take for my fibromyalgia? Why? Please explain how these drugs work.

Depending on your symptoms, their severity, and other medical conditions, your doctor can choose from various medications. Use this question to open a dialogue with your doctor about the best treatment combination for you.

The best answer to the "why?" question will be a full explanation that gives you the sense that your doctor has put thought into your personal case and isn't just giving you the same drugs she routinely prescribes for other fibromyalgia patients—or worse, because she doesn't believe in or understand fibromyalgia. You need to trust your doctor, but the savviest patients remain slightly skeptical. No one profits when you eat your vegetables or go to the gym, but both drug companies and some doctors earn money with prescriptions.

2. What percentage of improvement can I reasonably expect from this drug?

As you weigh the potential risks and benefits of taking any drug, hearing about the positive effects as a percentage may help clarify the facts. Ask your doctor to talk in specific terms, such as the average percentage of improvement for reducing sleep problems, pain, or fatigue.

No doctor can predict with absolute certainty how well a medication will help you, but this discussion establishes realistic expectations. Another big variable is your willingness to adopt healthier eating and exercise habits. Be sure your doctor explains your personal case and not just national averages.

3. How will you know if this drug is working well?

It's equally important to understand the details of how your doctor plans to assess and monitor a proposed drug's effectiveness over time, especially since fibromyalgia is a chronic disease without a cure.

Also ask, "How often will I need to make follow-up visits to the doctor's office or for laboratory tests?" and "How long will I have to take this drug for it to be effective?"

4. What short-term side effects are possible? Long-term side effects? Are there any side effects that may not go away?

Get the specifics on both short-term and long-term side effects. Be sure your doctor addresses this question for your specific case and not just with data from clinical trials or general studies.

Don't let your doctor gloss over his answer to this question. Double-check his response by searching the Internet for this medication by its generic and brand names. And don't forget to ask about potential permanent side effects and toxicity—a great question that few people think to ask.

5. How will you (the doctor) help me to manage any side effects?

This question will help you to learn more about side effects and if there are ways to lessen their impact on your health and well-being. For example, if you experience stomach upset, which is common with some medications, there may be simple over-the-counter remedies or another prescription to help control this problem.

6. What can *I* do to minimize the side effects and stay healthy?

Asking this question will help you feel like you are more in control of your own health. This question also implies that you and your doctor are a team, with both of you actively involved.

Sleep expert Dr. Charles R. Cantor at the University of Pennsylvania gives an example: "Some medications, including antidepressants, can improve sleep, but others cause insomnia. If your doctor doesn't know that your sleep quality is poor, he may not connect the dots between sleep problems and your antidepressant."

7. What, if any, restrictions will there be on my normal activities while I'm taking this drug?

Be sure you understand if there are any prohibitions on foods, other drugs, alcohol use, or any additional considerations you should know in advance. This is especially true if you still live a normal and active lifestyle, including travel, work, sex, sports, and outdoor activities.

8. What should I do if I miss a dose of my medicine?

Use your doctor's answer to solve any mysteries about whether or not you should double up or not in order to compensate for missed dosages.

9. What changes in my symptoms are serious enough for me to call you?

Find out the specifics about increased pain or disabling side effects.

Many people (especially women) hesitate to call their doctors for fear of "bothering" them or overreacting to new symptoms. Let your doctor's response guide you to a better-informed decision. If you aren't pleased with your doctor's response to this question, consider finding another one.

10. What is my overall treatment plan?

In addition to discussing specific drugs, you'll be smart to find out the big picture for your long-term care, treatment, and well-being. An overall treatment plan may include more tests, experiments with alternative therapies, lifestyle adjustments, and staying on top of breaking news about medical advances in fibromyalgia management.

Ask if the proposed treatment options will interfere with your other medications or will include lifestyle improvements (more exercise, better diet, etc.). Also clarify if you must take medications for the rest of your life and about your long-range chances for disability.

❯ The Magic Question

Are there less expensive medications for my fibromyalgia? Is there a generic version of this drug that is just as effective and cheaper?

Many people with a chronic illness like fibromyalgia have to take medications for an extended time. This is an important question to ask now as it could potentially save you hundreds or thousands of dollars.

Not all generic drugs are the same high-grade quality as their brand-name counterparts, so find out the specifics on the drugs your doctor is recommending for you.

Drug companies spend enormous amounts of money and effort to convince doctors and patients that their products are a worthy investment. With a diagnosis as frightening as fibromyalgia, you may not stop to consider, "What exactly am I putting in my body?" "Is it worth it?" "Is this drug a good value for my money?"

FOUR MORE TERRIFIC QUESTIONS

Sometimes 10 Best Questions just aren't enough. Ask these additional questions if they apply to your situation.

1. **Is there a drug I could try that might help more than just one symptom, like a drug for both pain and sleep disorders, or for pain and depression?**
   A smart strategy is to work with your doctor to find medications that you can tolerate and will serve dual purposes. This will help to minimize side effects, costs, and the amount of chemicals in your body.

2. **Are there any off-label medications that might help me?**
   The U.S. Food and Drug Administration allows doctors to prescribe approved medications for other uses, such as using the anticonvulsant drug Lyrica for pain relief. This is a common

practice, but your family physician may not be well informed or current on off-label options for fibromyalgia.

3. **Do you recommend that I retry a medication but with a different dosage?**
Fibromyalgia expert Dr. Kim Dupree Jones explains, "The drug companies' suggested dosages are sometimes not nearly the therapeutic dosage, so this explains why some patients think that a drug isn't working for them. It might be worth it to retry some of those drugs starting at a low dose and increasing slowly, to have much better outcomes." Dr. Patrick Wood says, "Fibromyalgia patients are frequently sensitive to medications, which their doctors are not aware of. Smaller (often tiny) doses may be effective."

4. **Do you ever prescribe placebos for your fibromyalgia patients?**
A 2008 study published in the *Journal of General Internal Medicine* reported that doctors commonly prescribe vitamins, over-the-counter pain killers, antibiotics, and sedatives to placate some patients. Ask this question (gently) if you suspect your doctor is not totally "fibro-friendly" or doesn't believe in your symptoms.

CONCLUSION

There is no single FDA-approved drug to prevent or relieve all the symptoms of fibromyalgia. Any ongoing drug regimen should be administered in combination with a proactive approach to adopting a healthier lifestyle (see part 3) and an open mind about alternative therapies (chapters 9 and 10).

Use your doctor's advice and answers to make a better-informed decision about the drugs that he is recommending for you. If you are still unsure about what to do, ask your doctor this follow-up question: "If you were making this decision for your sister or a loved one with symptoms like mine, what would you do?"

Consider your personal priorities and financial situation as you *ask yourself* these two additional questions: "Are these drugs cost effective for me?" "Will they improve my quality of life?"

Everyone's fibromyalgia symptoms and life situations are different, so there are no right or wrong answers. Some people are happy for any slight improvement, while others dismiss small improvements as insufficient to justify the costs or hassle. Your quality-of-life issues are an important consideration as you and your doctor evaluate what's best for you.

THE 10 BEST RESOURCES

About.com. "Fibromyalgia Medications." http://arthritis.about.com/od/ fmsmeds/Fibromyalgia_Medications_Fibromyalgia_Drugs_Fibromyalgia_ Medicines.htm.

Arthritis Foundation. "Fibromyalgia (FMS): Treatment Options." www .arthritis.org/disease-center.php?disease_id=10&df=treatments.

Consumers Reports Health.org. "Anticonvulsants Drugs: Summary of Recommendations." www.consumerreports.org/health/best-buy-drugs/anticonvulsants.htm.

Drugs.com. "Fibromyalgia." www.drugs.com/search.php?searchterm= Fibromyalgia&is_main_search=1&type=1.

Fibromyalgia Symptoms.org. "Fibromyalgia Medications." www .fibromyalgia-symptoms.org/fibromyalgia-medications.html.

IGuard.org. "Drug Search." http://iguard.org.

Medicare. "Medicare Prescription Drug Plan Finder." www.medicare.gov.

MedlinePlus. "Drugs, Supplements, and Herbal Information." (Search by drug name.) www.nlm.nih.gov/medlineplus/druginformation.html.

U.S. Food and Drug Administration. "Information about the Products We Regulate." www.fda.gov/cder/drug/default.htm.

U.S. Food and Drug Administration. "Living with Fibromyalgia, Drugs Approved to Manage Pain." www.fda.gov/consumer/updates/ fibromyalgia062107.html.

CHAPTER 9

THE 10 BEST QUESTIONS

For Choosing Alternative Therapies for
Fibromyalgia

Turn your wounds into wisdom.

—Oprah Winfrey

The term **alternative medicine** (also called **alternative treatments** or **alternative therapies**) describes any healing practice that is outside the boundaries of conventional Western medicine. Common examples include dietary supplements, meditation, naturopathy, herbals, yoga, hypnosis, and chiropractic treatments. Alternative treatments are often used *instead of* conventional medicine (such as acupuncture to replace pain medications).

In contrast, **complementary medicine** or **complementary treatments** are used *together* with conventional medicine (such as therapeutic massage used along with a prescription pain medication). The umbrella term is **complementary and alternative medicine (CAM)**. The term **integrative medicine** describes a combination of conventional and CAM therapies.

In reality, all of these terms are often used interchangeably, although some medical professionals prefer clear distinctions. The definitions are constantly changing as yesterday's CAM treatment proves safe and effective enough to become today's mainstream medicine. (Here the terms are used interchangeably, too.)

Dr. Mimi Guarneri, the medical director of the Scripps Center for Integrative Medicine in La Jolla, California, further explains, "CAM applies to treatment modalities not taught in Western medicine. Our goal is to use global healing traditions that are evidence-based and enhance the practice of conventional medicine."

Alternative therapies for fibromyalgia abound because there are no fool-proof medications or treatments in conventional medicine. The good news is that there are many alternative pain treatments you can experiment with that are relatively risk free, low or no cost, and work for some patients.

The bad news is that in the vacuum of standardized fibromyalgia diagnostic tools and treatments and the lack of federal guidelines a huge market of bogus treatments has sprung up. There are many clever people who make a very good living preying on fibromyalgia patients with phony products and services. See more in chapter 10.

Ask your doctor these following Best Questions to seek his blessing prior to starting an alternative therapy.

THE QUESTION DOCTOR SAYS:

Check out appealing CAM options before your doctor appointment so that you'll be ready to ask your own specific questions on a particular alternative therapy.

>>> THE 10 BEST QUESTIONS
For Choosing Alternative Therapies for Fibromyalgia

1. Do you think I'm a good candidate for alternative therapies? Why or why not?

Perhaps the most important aspect of this discussion with your doctor is that you are having it at all. Not many patients who use alternative therapies talk with their doctors about them. Sometimes doctors lack in-depth knowledge about CAM.

Dr. Brent A. Bauer, the Director of the Complementary and Integrative Medicine Program at the Mayo Clinic, explains, "I find that most conventionally trained physicians are increasingly open to discussing various CAM or integrative treatments. They may not always have a full understanding of the therapy, but most are aware that there has been a significant growth in both the volume and the quality of research in this area."

This question is important to ensure that a CAM treatment (such as supplements) won't interfere with conventional treatment (such as prescription drugs). Dr. Jessica Black, a naturopathic physician in Oregon, advises, "You might be wasting your money on supplements if your body can't absorb these vitamins."

If your doctor doesn't believe you are a good candidate and you are still interested, ask if you could try an alternative therapy later. There may be good reasons for your doctor's hesitation.

2. Which alternative therapies do you recommend for me for relief from my physical symptoms? Why?

An easy classification system divides CAM treatments into two classes: passive and active. A **passive therapy** is one where someone does something to you, such as a massage or acupuncture. An **active therapy** is one where you are the main actor, like attending a yoga class or praying.

Both passive and active therapies can ease fibromyalgia symptoms. Be sure you understand your doctor's rationale as well as her specific recommendations for you.

Dr. Daniel J. Clauw, a fibromyalgia expert at the University of Michigan, says, "Most of them [CAM therapies] haven't been well studied so it is difficult to know exactly 'what works.' But most of these treatments are safe and worth trying especially if individuals haven't responded to other treatments."

Fibromyalgia expert Dr. Michael McNett adds, "If your doctor is familiar with and not automatically against any over-the-counter products, don't be shy about asking about them."

Think outside the box, too. As Australian fibromyalgia sufferer Dot Gerecke says, "For me, piano is therapy. I can forget everything else, even pain, if it isn't too bad. I also believe having a pet is very important. Even on bad days, you have to get out of bed to care and feed your pet. My black Labrador, Mica, was my guardian and companion."

3. Which alternative therapies do you recommend to help me with emotional or psychological issues? Please explain your rationale.

Dr. Herbert Benson, author of the best-selling book, *The Relaxation Response,* and a noted mind-body expert, says, "People have anxieties regardless of how life-threatening their disease is."

Ask specifically about alternative therapies to ease your depression, stress, or anxiety. Alternative therapies aim to balance the whole person—physically, mentally, and emotionally—while standard pain treatments are doing their job.

Dr. Kim Dupree Jones, a fibromyalgia expert at the Oregon Health & Science University, explains, "Complementary and alternative therapies are sometimes better as add-on therapies rather than first-line therapies."

Again, make sure you understand why your doctor has recommended this therapy and how long you should continue it.

4. What benefits or improvements can I reasonably expect from these therapies?

Your doctor may not know because there is still so much that isn't well understood about either CAM treatments or fibromyalgia.

Seattle-based fibromyalgia expert, Dr. Patrick Wood, says,

"Well-researched and rationally targeted alternative therapies can be very beneficial. The movement therapies like yoga and tai chi should be considered. Although they have not been proven to reduce pain, they can play an important role in conditioning the patient for aerobic exercise which is really critical."

The medical community has only recently become interested in alternative treatments, so this means there aren't as many evidence-based studies as for conventional treatments, especially with fibromyalgia. To see alternative treatment clinical trials for fibromyalgia, click on fibromyalgia at www.clinicaltrials.gov.

5. Are there any potential side effects or dangers if I use alternative treatments?

There is a wide range of possible side effects across the highly diverse spectrum of alternative treatments. Regardless of the treatment, you want one that's both safe and effective.

Some therapies are no-risk therapies, including prayer and meditation techniques. Other therapies have some risks, such as massages, acupuncture, or yoga practice.

Ask your doctor if there are treatment standards or guidelines for the recommended alternative treatments you're considering. Also discuss your other medical conditions or any previous injuries.

6. In your opinion, do the known benefits outweigh the risks for this therapy?

If the answer is no, explore your doctor's rationale.

7. Are there any alternative treatments that I should totally avoid?

Some supplements, herbs, or other treatments can interfere with your conventional treatments. You may be easily injured with some forms of alternative therapy.

Keep in mind the difference between treatments that *add* to conventional therapies and ones that *replace* conventional therapies. See chapter 10 on bogus treatments to avoid.

8. Should I let you know before I start an alternative treatment?

This question serves to give you the official stamp of approval on your choices. Also ask about your doctor's preference for staying informed during the duration of your alternative treatments. You might not want to report every yoga class to your doctor, but give him the option of stating his preferred protocol.

9. What's the best way to find a certified practitioner or learn more about alternative treatments?

Once you have an alternative treatment plan, you'll need a well-qualified practitioner. Rather than holding an M.D. degree (medical doctor), the practitioners are usually naturopaths, physical therapists, psychologists, physiatrists (rehabilitation specialists), and other health care professionals.

Ask a practitioner if he is licensed by a credible institution. Look up this institution on the Internet to make sure it's legitimate. Ask if he belongs to a national association in his field. Ask how many years total experience he has and how many fibromyalgia patients he's treated in the past.

Interview the practitioner in advance and make sure you feel comfortable. Shop around if needed. Your doctor, support group, or friends can give you referrals. See chapters 12 and 13 for choosing a massage therapist or acupuncturist.

10. Will this therapy be covered by my insurance?

Alternative treatments run the gamut from free to pricey. Your health insurance provider may not cover the cost or only offer partial coverage. If your doctor or her office staff can't help you with this question, check directly with your insurance company to clarify your coverage before you start any costly CAM treatments.

❯ The Magic Question

What's the latest reading you've done on CAM or alternative therapies for fibromyalgia?

This question will help you understand your doctor's own personal interest, knowledge, and possible biases about alternative treatments. The reality is that CAM is hot in many medical circles, but not all doctors are equally knowledgeable or tuned in.

A lot of CAM isn't rocket science but just down-to-earth strategies for a healthier lifestyle and a preventive care mind-set. Your doctor will be somewhere along a continuum of involvement with CAM.

It makes good sense to understand if your doctor is a CAM skeptic or cheerleader. If you feel strongly about wanting a better CAM cheerleader, use chapters 2, 3, and 4 for guidance.

PRIMER ON TYPES OF ALTERNATIVE THERAPIES FOR FIBROMYALGIA

The National Center for Complementary and Alternative Medicine states that 90 percent of people with fibromyalgia use some type of CAM. These practices and their effectiveness vary widely. Examples include:

❯ Massage therapy and oriental medicine — See chapter 12 for more details.

❯ Acupuncture — See chapter 13 for more details.

❯ Prayer and meditation — See chapter 27 for more details.

❯ Yoga and tai chi — Helps pain with gentle, slow movements.

> Water exercise — Move in warm water, swim, or take a water aerobics class.

> Physical therapy — Get professional help through movement exercises.

> Biofeedback — Uses electronics to control your responses to stress and pain.

> Chiropractic care — Eases back pain and may increase pain tolerance.

> Herbal remedies — Improves sleep disturbances (supplements such as valerian root extracts) and other symptoms.

> Natural dietary supplements — Relieves symptoms through magnesium, melatonin, acetyl-L-carnitine, SAM-e, probiotics, and others.

> Hypnosis — Reduces pain using professional or self-hypnosis.

> Magnet therapy — Uses magnetic energy to promote healing.

> Pet ownership — Care for a pet as a therapeutic outlet.

> Music and art therapy — Create and relax with either a paint brush or piano.

CONCLUSION

The effectiveness of many CAM treatments is still unknown. Mayo Clinic's Dr. Bauer says, "Realize that there is no 'silver bullet' or 'one-size-fits-all' cure for fibromyalgia. Each person with fibromyalgia is unique."

Rosie Hamlin, famous for her 1960s hit song, "Angel Baby," and a fibromyalgia sufferer, advises, "I think a person needs to find out what is the best thing that helps you. I went to acupuncture, water therapy, and tai chi. I tried everything. Water therapy helped me a lot."

Virginia-based information systems engineer and fibromyalgia patient Abby MacLean agrees, "My advice is to keep looking for the alternative therapy that works for you. There's no one right thing for everybody. Keep an open mind and if one thing doesn't work, be willing to try something else."

THE 10 BEST RESOURCES

American Pain Foundation. "Complementary/Alternative Medicine Articles & Web Links." www.painfoundation.org/page.asp?file=Links/CAM.htm.

Hammerly, Milton. *Fibromyalgia—The New Integrative Approach: How to Combine the Best of Traditional and Alternative Therapies.* Cincinnati, OH: Adams Media, 1997.

Kabat-Zinn, Jon. *Wherever You Go, There You Are: Mindfulness Meditation in Everyday Life,* 10th ed. New York: Hyperion, 2005.

National Center for Complementary and Alternative Medicine. "All NCCAM Clinical Trials." (Choose fibromyalgia.) http://nccam.nih.gov/clinicaltrials/alltrials.htm.

National Center for Complementary and Alternative Medicine. "CAM and Fibromyalgia: At a Glance." http://nccam.nih.gov/news/newsletter/2008_july/fibromyalgia.htm.

National Fibromyalgia Association. "Alternative Treatment Options for Fibromyalgia." www.fmaware.org/site/News2?page=NewsArticle&id=6135.

National Fibromyalgia Association. "Successfully Working with PT and OT." www.fmaware.org/site/News2?page=NewsArticle&id=6160.

National Fibromyalgia Association. "Thoughts on a New Integrative Approach." www.fmaware.org/site/News2?page=NewsArticle&id=5233.

Siegel, Bernie S. *Love, Medicine and Miracles: Lessons Learned about Self-Healing from a Surgeon's Experience with Exceptional Patients.* New York: Harper Paperbacks, 1990.

Weil, Andrew. *Natural Health, Natural Medicine: The Complete Guide to Wellness and Self-Care for Optimum Health,* revised ed. Boston: Houghton Mifflin, 2004.

CHAPTER 10: THE 10 BEST QUESTIONS

To Avoid Being Scammed

Precaution is better than cure.

—Johann Wolfgang Goethe

You may not realize it, but you are exceedingly vulnerable to losing a wad of money to a con artist specializing in bogus alternative fibromyalgia treatments. The U.S. Department of Health and Human Services, the Federal Trade Commission, and the U.S. Food and Drug Administration all warn that because fibromyalgia has no clearly superior treatments, some desperate patients are easily tempted to try unproven, unscientific, and sometimes dangerous treatments.

You are like a dinner bell to con artists promoting dubious supplements, herbs, and pain management devices. These unscrupulous snake oil salesmen know how to prey on your pain, emotions, and fears.

Even if you think you are too savvy to get scammed, there are many slick Web sites with impressive sounding medical lingo, big promises, and endless testimonials from "happily cured" patients that might sound too tempting. As Dr. Stephen Barrett, founder of the consumer watchdog Web site, Quackwatch, warns, "Don't let desperation cloud your judgment."

Ask yourself the following Best Questions to make objective decisions about questionable CAM treatments. Talk with your doctor if you are unsure about trying an advertised alternative treatment.

> **THE QUESTION DOCTOR SAYS:**
>
> You can also easily tailor these Best Questions to ask during a telephone sales call, about television infomercials, or when talking with a salesman face to face about products and services.

>>> THE 10 BEST QUESTIONS
To Avoid Being Scammed

1. Who's behind this claim or alternative treatment?

Any Web site or company offering medical treatments should offer responsible people's names and their medical credentials. Even if someone sounds impressive, search the Internet for his name and articles in professional medical journals. Run the other way as fast as you can if no one is home at this Web site or company.

2. Are the people offering the alternative treatments also the same people who are selling them?

The funding sources behind this Web site should be clearly explained. Information from a neutral or disinterested third party is usually more reliable than information from someone who benefits personally from product sales.

3. Does this treatment offer a cure, remission, or healing?

Alternative treatments for fibromyalgia include high-dose vitamin supplements, diets, herbal remedies, gadgets, and dietary practices like detoxification. Not all are bad for you or bogus, but some are potentially harmful.

Avoid Web sites with flowery medical jargon, claims to cure fibromyalgia (impossible), and multiple ads on the Web site, especially money-back guarantees or free trials. Read these Web sites carefully several times or ask for a trusted friend's opinion.

Concerns about alternative drugs or supplements include:

- Unknown effectiveness or safety
- Unknown purity
- No monitoring of bad reactions
- Can interfere with prescription drugs

4. Does the Web site or company have a seal of credibility?

If the Web site or company does not have an approval or accreditation seal that doesn't automatically make it bogus. But a seal of credibility may provide a measure of quality assurance. Check with Health on the Net (www.hon.ch) and URAC (www.urac.org) to verify seals.

5. Is this alternative treatment offered as a "miracle" cure?

Look out for phrases like "scientific breakthrough," "miraculous cure," "secret ingredient," or "ancient remedy." Don't believe claims that the therapy has "endured for decades or centuries" or that there are many "testimonials" claiming phenomenal success rates. Beware of extravagant claims using words like *always* or *never.*

6. Are any prior studies offered as scientific evidence, or are there only anecdotal stories and personal testimonials to back up the claimed benefits of this alternative treatment?

You want specific scientific evidence including measurable results in hard, cold numbers, not that fibromyalgia patient "Kathleen" in Houston loves the taste and won an Olympic gold medal in gymnastics afterwards.

7. What other documentation is given to support the Web site's or company's claims?

Look for more information, especially in established medical journals, not e-magazines or blogs. Be wary of listings that are old or stopped being updated more than a year ago.

8. Does this alternative treatment or company claim to have exclusive rights to the treatments offered?

Real treatments have well-documented studies with hundreds or thousands of patients. Fake treatments are available from only one doctor, clinic, or Web site. It doesn't make sense that there would be a monopoly on new products or treatments as good as these.

9. Has any conventional medical organization endorsed this product or treatment?

Endorsements by trusted names in medical science and rheumatology are a good sign. In contrast, scammers emphasize that others—usually highly respected doctors or "the establishment"—are trying to suppress the distribution of their products.

10. Is personal information or money requested up front?

Avoid Web sites that won't tell you anything until you've created an account with them and revealed your name, e-mail address, credit card number, or other personal details. Red flags include requests for money up front or perpetual discounts, like "40 percent off."

❯ The Magic Question

If a medical breakthrough really had occurred for fibromyalgia, would the news be announced first in an ad?

The credit for this common-sense Magic Question belongs to the Federal Trade Commission, the federal government's consumer watchdog organization. The con artists' claim of "exclusive rights" is the ultimate tip-off that you are dealing with bogus treatments.

Dr. Patrick Wood, a Seattle-based fibromyalgia expert, warns, "There's a lot of snake oil that falls under the label of alternative medicine. The ones that promise fibromyalgia cure-all in fifteen days are a lot of phooey."

CONCLUSION

According to the National Institutes of Health, about 62 percent of all people with serious illnesses try alternative therapies. The effectiveness of many CAM therapies is still unknown. In contrast, bogus health companies aim for your vulnerabilities—and your wallet.

Mayo Clinic's director of the Complementary and Integrative Medicine Program, Dr. Brent A. Bauer, says, "Homework! This means that we must do some investigation before we invest our scarce resources in something that sounds too good to be true."

Oregon-based fibromyalgia expert Dr. Kim Dupree Jones concludes, "Unfortunately, there's a fair amount of quackery in fibromyalgia treatments. Any infomercial that you see at two o'clock in the morning that says it's for fibromyalgia and baldness is not a product you want to try."

THE 10 BEST RESOURCES

Federal Citizen Information Center. "State, County and City Government Consumer Protection Offices." www.consumeraction.gov/state.shtml.

Federal Trade Commission. "Virtual 'Treatments' Can Be Real-World Deceptions." www.ftc.gov/bcp/conline/pubs/alerts/mrclalrt.shtm.

Health on the Net Foundation. "HONcode Site Evaluation Form." www .hon.ch/HONcode/HONcode_check.html.

National Institute on Aging. "Health Quackery: Spotting Health Scams." www.nia.nih.gov/HealthInformation/Publications/quackery.htm.

National Institute on Aging. "Online Health Information: Can You Trust It?" www.nia.nih.gov/HealthInformation/Publications/onlinehealth.htm.

Quackwatch, operated by Barrett, Stephen, and Victor Herbert. "Twenty-Five Ways to Spot Quacks and Vitamin Pushers." www.quackwatch .com/01QuackeryRelatedTopics/spotquack.html.

U.S. Administration on Aging. "Consumer Protection Tips." www.aoa .gov/smp/consprof/consprof_resources_tips.asp.

U.S. Food and Drug Administration. "2008 Safety Alerts for Drugs, Biologics, Medical Devices, and Cosmetics." www.fda.gov/medwatch/ safety/2008/safety08.htm.

U.S. Food and Drug Administration. "Buying Prescription Medicine Online: A Consumer Safety Guide." www.fda.gov/cder/consumerinfo/ buyOnlineGuide_text.htm.

URAC. "Consumer Resource Center." www.urac.org/consumers/resources.

Before Participating in a Clinical Trial

> Today, only a small percentage of consumers are aware of clinical trials as a health-care option, both from a standpoint of receiving a high level of care and in helping develop the latest products to treat debilitating or life-threatening diseases.
>
> —Dr. C. Everett Koop, former U.S. Surgeon General,
> during a 2006 interview with the author

A *clinical trial* (also called a "clinical study") is a research program conducted with patients to evaluate a new medical treatment or drug. For example, there are clinical trials with people who have fibromyalgia to search for causes, better drugs, and more useful alternative therapies. Clinical trials make the newest scientific advances possible. Yesterday's clinical trial is today's newest fibromyalgia drug.

In 2004, more than 2 million people in the United States volunteered for industry- and government-sponsored studies (for all diseases). There are more than eighty thousand clinical trials in the United States annually and the numbers are growing.

Because fibromyalgia treatment is complex, it's not likely that a breakthrough cure will be discovered in any one given clinical trial. If you are interested in participating, just be realistic that a miracle cure isn't likely to be discovered during your clinical trial. Every study and person involved matters, but research usually progresses from small steps and many studies.

Sometimes people make hasty or poorly informed decisions.

According to a 2002 study by CenterWatch, a leading authority on clinical trials, 70 percent of the volunteers entering
clinical trials didn't know what questions to ask before the trial
started. Many people reported that they didn't understand the
risks of their participation, and 10 percent of the volunteers
admitted they didn't read the informed consent form before
signing it.

There are two lists of 10 Best Questions in this chapter. Ask
your doctor the first set of Best Questions for factual information.
Ask yourself the second list of Best Questions to decide if a clinical
trial is right for you. These questions should not replace medical
advice.

>>> THE 10 BEST QUESTIONS
Before Participating in a Clinical Trial

1. How will this trial help me personally?

Keep this conversation at the personal level—the benefits for you
personally—rather than generic or statistical facts. Your bottom-
line question is, "What's in it for me?" Be sure you understand
how your clinical trial treatments will differ from more conventional treatment.

The benefits of participating in a clinical trial may include:

- Increased patient monitoring by a medical team and generally a higher standard of care
- Possible health care benefits, such as free genetic tests for
  family members
- The opportunity to help others who suffer from
  fibromyalgia

2. What are the researchers hoping to learn from this study? What phase is this trial?

Clinical trials are developed for different reasons. Some study the effectiveness of certain drugs while others study safe dosages. Know the exact purpose of the study prior to signing on.

A key follow-up question to ask is, "What phase is this trial?" Clinical trials are usually conducted in a series of steps, called Phase I, Phase II, Phase III, and Phase IV trials.

- **Phase I** trials enroll limited numbers of volunteers in limited locations to assess drug tolerance, safety, side effects, and risks.
- **Phase II** trials study the effectiveness of a new drug in different doses in a few hundred volunteers with this condition.
- **Phase III** trials use many volunteers and provide the main evidence for the U.S. Food and Drug Administration's (FDA) decisions to approve or reject this new drug.
- **Phase IV** trials use large numbers of volunteers to further evaluate a drug's long-term safety and effectiveness after FDA approval.

3. Who is sponsoring this trial? Describe this trial's prior history and measurable outcomes.

This important question aims to understand more about the researchers' motives. The gold standard in clinical trials is sponsorship by a highly respected organization such as the National Institutes of Health. Drug companies can also offer solid and ethical trials but usually also hope to earn megabucks from a breakthrough new drug. By understanding the trial's sponsors, you'll have clues into their possible biases. See the Magic Question below.

Ask your doctor "who, what, when, where, and why" questions to prompt a full explanation from him. Find out if you'll be required to switch doctors or care centers. You don't necessarily want to be seen by a series of rotating doctors, each one being another "get acquainted" chore for you.

4. What are the possible risks and complications, both short term and long term, in my case?

Most trials are safe but there may be some risks. CenterWatch found that one in thirty volunteers typically experiences a serious side effect, and one in ten thousand dies as a result of the effects of a study drug.

Potential risks include:

- It is possible that the experimental drug is inferior to current standard treatments.
- You may be randomly assigned to the **placebo drug** that is inactive.
- The experimental drug may not work for you personally.
- There may be long-term residual effects from the trial's drug.
- Your health insurance carrier may not cover all study costs.
- Some trials are time consuming or disruptive to daily routines.

A really smart follow-up question is, "What *don't* we know yet about this new drug or treatment?" This question will encourage your doctor to reveal more candidly any design flaws and possible side effects. If your doctor doesn't know this answer, ask him how you can find out.

4. What safety measures are built into this study?

Your doctor's answer should include details about patient safeguards and patient safety monitoring.

Ask, "Has this study been approved by an **institutional review board** (an ethical panel comprised of doctors and other medical experts who work with the FDA)?" and "Did the review board have any ethical concerns with the trial?" Also ask about how your personal and medical information will be protected from identity theft or other unauthorized disclosures.

5. How long will this trial last? Where is it being conducted?

The length of clinical trials varies greatly, as does the amount of time required of you on a daily, weekly, or monthly basis. Know the expected duration of your trial before signing on.

Be sure to find out the total time the trial will last (in days, weeks, months, or years). Then ask "How often?" and "How long?" to gauge your time commitment on a routine basis (daily or monthly).

Don't get caught off guard about the location of the trial. Ask if you'll have to travel to another town to participate.

7. What kind of support will I receive during the trial?

Find out in advance what your insurance carrier will cover and what costs will come out of your own pocket. Also don't forget incidental costs, like additional child care, time off from work, or gas money. Ask if you'll be compensated either by your insurance carrier or the study's sponsors. The sponsors may offer partial payment of your medical expenses as part of the study. But be skeptical at first and find out (in writing) exactly who pays for what.

Ask, "Who will be on my medical team?" "Who can I call if I have questions?" "Who will be in charge of my care during the trial, especially if I experience side effects?" and "Who will cover costs if I have complications or serious side effects from this trial?"

8. What will happen when the trial ends?

Be sure you understand what kind of support (if any) you can expect after the trial ends. Will you receive medical care or some other kind of support follow-up care?

Ask, "Will I have any post-trial responsibilities?" and "Who will be responsible for the post-trial segment of this study?"

Sometimes the new drug or treatment is so useful that participants want to continue with it even after the trial ends. Find out if this will be an option for you. Ask, "Can I opt to remain on this treatment even after termination of the trial?" "Will I have to pay for medications to continue, and if so, how much will it cost?"

Lastly, you probably will want to know about how the study turned out. Find out how you will get the results at the trial's conclusion.

9. What happens if I'm harmed by the trial? Can I freely withdraw at any time without penalty?

Don't neglect to examine the worst-case scenario about patient safety. Ask, "What will happen?" "Who will be responsible and accountable?" and "Who will pay for my medical expenses if I'm injured?"

Ask about the conditions and provisions for withdrawal. Your informed consent form should spell out an escape clause. Clarify if you can quit the trial at any time without consequences. If you leave early, find out if you'll have to seek treatment elsewhere and if there will be any restrictions on your future treatments. Sometimes a volunteer must leave the study early due to a change in his or her health status that makes it dangerous or difficult to participate.

10. Am I a good candidate? Why or why not? What is your recommendation?

Ask your doctor to summarize this discussion and state if you are a good candidate, both from a medical perspective and in terms of eligibility.

Stay alert to any possible bias on your doctor's part due to her own participation in a certain trial. You can phrase the question as something like, "If you weren't doing this research, what would you say is best for me?" If you feel pressured to participate, get an objective second opinion (see chapter 5).

AM I RIGHT FOR A CLINICAL TRIAL?

Before volunteering for a clinical trial assess your readiness and willingness to be a guinea pig.

1. **What are my personal goals for wanting to participate in a clinical trial?** Be very honest with yourself about your own motivations. Seriously consider your available time and energy and how debilitating your symptoms and pain are before you sign up.
2. **How far am I willing to go?** Examine your tolerance for taking risks.
3. **Do I have the time needed to participate in a clinical trial?** Some clinical trials are time consuming and may take years, while others are much shorter.
4. **How important is it to me that I work with my current doctor?** If your current doctor is not part of the clinical trial, you may need to find a new doctor who is.
5. **Am I confident and comfortable with the goals of this study and with the staff at the research center?** Ideally, the trial's goals match your personal values and the staff will treat you well.

6. **How important is it to me to help other people with fibromyalgia?** Participating in a clinical trial is a way of helping future generations of fibromyalgia patients if this is your thing.

7. **How will this trial affect my daily life?** Logistical concerns include travel time and expenses, child care needs, and time off from work.

8. **Will my family support my decision to participate in this clinical trial?** Talk this over with the other people in your life who will be affected.

9. **Have I read the informed consent document and taken enough time to truly understand it? Has everything been adequately explained to me?** Be sure to ask about anything that's unclear to you, especially about any confusing fine print.

10. **How realistic am I about what I have to gain personally from participating?** Answer this question after you've done your homework.

THE QUESTION DOCTOR SAYS:

Ask lots of questions before you sign anything, especially about the fine print in the informed consent document. These documents can be confusing for even the most intelligent people.

❯ The Magic Question

Does my doctor or the study sponsor have a strong bias favoring my participation?

Doctors and research centers recommend specific clinical trials for a variety of reasons. While most are for humanitarian and scientific motives, there are a few exceptions.

Some doctors are paid by drug companies to recruit their patients into clinical trials. Drug companies want to move newly approved drugs quickly to the marketplace, especially for potential high-profit earners like new medicines for fibromyalgia. Other doctors gain professional prestige by being involved and publishing trial results in medical journals.

If you suspect your doctor is pushing you, ask her directly, "Do you have anything to gain from my participation in this clinical trial?" This is your "better safe than sorry" question before participating in a clinical trial.

CONCLUSION

You want to fully understand exactly what you're getting into ahead of time if you choose to participate in a clinical trial. Each person's experience in a clinical trial is unique.

Fibromyalgia research is currently at a special crossroads, somewhere between medical scorn and gaining full acceptance as a "real disease." As Dr. Patrick Wood, a fibromyalgia expert in Seattle, observes, "Having pharmaceutical companies take an interest is going to change the landscape, but we are still 'waiting for Prozac' in the fibromyalgia world. There's still the need for a magic bullet for fibromyalgia like Prozac has been for depression."

Remember, participation in a clinical trial is always voluntary. These Best Questions will help you decide if you want to be a guinea pig for science—or not.

THE 10 BEST RESOURCES

Center for Information and Study on Clinical Research Participation. "Education Before Participation." www.ciscrp.org/information/documents/ 2006BrochureEnglish.pdf.

Centerwatch.com. Lists more than 41,000 trials mainly conducted by the pharmaceutical industry. Search by therapeutic category or condition. www.centerwatch.com.

ClinicalTrials.gov. A comprehensive registry of federally and privately supported clinical trials in the United States and worldwide. http://clinicaltrials.gov.

ClinicalTrials.gov. "Understanding Clinical Trials." www.clinicaltrials.gov/ct2/info/understand.

ECRI. "Should I Enter a Clinical Trial? A Patient Reference Guide for Adults with a Serious or Life-Threatening Illness." www.ecri.org/Documents/Clinical_Trials_Patient_Reference_Guide.pdf.

Getz, Ken, and Deborah Borfitz. *Informed Consent: The Consumer's Guide to the Risks and Benefits of Volunteering for Clinical Trials.* Boston: CenterWatch, 2002.

National Fibromyalgia Association. "Listing of Current Clinical Trials." www.fmaware.org/site/PageServer?pagename=research_clinicalTrials.

National Fibromyalgia Association. "Research Overview." www.fmaware.org/site/PageServer?pagename=research_overview.

National Fibromyalgia Association. "What Are Clinical Trials and Why You Should Volunteer." www.fmaware.org/site/PageServer?pagename=research_clinicalTrialsParticipation.

Wikipedia. "Clinical Trial." http://en.wikipedia.org/wiki/clinical_trial.

CHAPTER 12: THE 10 BEST QUESTIONS
To Find a Great Massage Therapist

Often the hands will solve a mystery that the intellect has struggled with in vain.

—Carl G. Jung

Some people find tremendous relief in massage therapy as an alternative treatment for their fibromyalgia symptoms. A **massage** is the systematic manual application of pressure and movement to the body's soft tissues. There are literally hundreds of different types of massage called **modalities**, including the most common type, Swedish massage.

Research studies on pain relief through massage, such as a 2002 fibromyalgia study by Touch Research Institute in Miami, have confirmed positive results along with improved sleep and decreased depression. Benefits vary widely depending on the massage therapist's skill, techniques, and choice of modalities.

The president of the American Massage Therapy Association, M. K. Brennan, says, "Just like every massage is going to be felt differently by different people, every massage therapist has a different personality. You want to find a massage therapist that you feel you can communicate well with."

Even a little relief can mean a lot. Studies indicate that the feel-good neurotransmitters serotonin and dopamine spike with a good massage. However, many fibromyalgia experts and patients also caution that a deep, vigorous, or overly long massage can worsen fibromyalgia symptoms or cause a flare-up.

For example, Virginia fibromyalgia patient Abby MacLean cautions, "I think you have to be very careful even if they are licensed.

If you have a big, whopping knot in your muscle, pressing down hard may initially relieve it, but the rebound can cause tremendous damage."

The smartest way to protect your body and your wallet when you are looking for a quality massage is to ask the following Best Questions. Use your doctor, fibromyalgia support group, family, or friends to generate a list of their favorite massage therapists you can call. Check in advance with your health insurance provider about coverage.

THE QUESTION DOCTOR SAYS:

If you are naturally shy, have little previous experience with massages, or worry about your appearance, see the 10 Most Embarrassing Questions (and answers), page 116.

>>> THE 10 BEST QUESTIONS
To Find a Great Massage Therapist

1. Are you licensed to practice massage in this state?

Forty-one states regulate the massage therapy profession with licenses, registrations, or certification requirements. See more at the American Massage Therapy Association's Web site at www .amtamassage.org/about/lawstate.html. Some local governments also have regulations.

2. Do you have a business license? Do you work in a business-like setting?

Don't confuse a standard business license, which is required of anyone operating a small business, with a professional massage license. Your massage therapist should have both.

She should also give massages in a professional, business-like setting even if she performs massages in her home. There should be a private room used for massages only with a professional massage table, equipment, and soft lighting.

M. K. Brennan advises, "If a massage therapist seems too open to seeing you anytime or anyplace, you might think twice. You want a business professional." If in doubt, ask to see her business license.

3. Are you a current member of the American Massage Therapy Association (AMTA)?

Professional members of AMTA have demonstrated their competency through successful completion of the National Certification Exam offered by the National Certification Board of Therapeutic Massage and Bodywork or graduation from an accredited program. Members must also pursue continuing education in order to retain membership. There are approximately fifty-eight thousand members.

There are other professional associations, including the American Medical Massage Association and the International Massage Association, but AMTA membership is the gold standard.

4. Are you certified by the National Certification Board of Therapeutic Massage and Bodywork (NCBTMB)?

Massage professionals earn this nationally recognized certification by mastering core massage techniques, passing a standardized exam, abiding by the NCBTMB's ethical code, taking continuing education programs, and reestablishing their credentials every four years.

These high standards are your best protection. But only about one-third of U.S. massage therapists have this optional credential. See the NCBTMB Web site to find a certified massage therapist near you (www.ncbtmb.org/consumers_find_practitioner.php).

5. Where did you receive your massage therapy training? Did you graduate from a program accredited by the Commission on Massage Therapy Accreditation (COMTA)?

Proper training by qualified faculty is essential. Find the directory of COMTA's recognized schools and educational programs at their Web site (www.comta.org/directory.php).

6. How many hours of initial training did you have? How long have you been doing massages?

The AMTA recommends at least five hundred hours of training. This is also the standard for many states that regulate massage therapists. Some college education is a good sign.

While some new therapists are excellent, look for a massage therapist with more than three years experience. M. K. Brennan says this is when massage therapists most frequently leave the profession for professional and personal reasons.

If this massage therapist hesitates or waffles on answers, be at least a little suspicious. These are basic and fair questions.

7. Are you trained in any specific massage modalities?

Each modality requires specialized training. You really need someone who is focused on pain relief.

For fibromyalgia, the very best answer to this question is training in neuromuscular or trigger point therapy, and/or myofascial release techniques. The AMTA offers specific continuing education in fibromyalgia. At minimum, you want a therapist whose style is long, soothing strokes coupled with friction strokes over muscle knots to release toxins and pain.

M. K. Brennan advises, "Most massage therapists have a 'tool bag' of various techniques they mix and match to adapt to a client's needs. It's important to ask, 'What can you do and how does that apply to me?'"

8. How many other clients with chronic pain have you massaged? How many of these are ongoing clients?

Asking these two questions will help you gauge this massage therapist's experience and knowledge of fibromyalgia. Ideally, he will have learned techniques by working on others with fibromyalgia and you won't be his guinea pig.

Finding out about this person's rate of return clients can be a big clue to how satisfied others have been. If he doesn't have experience with chronic pain clients, a good follow-up question is, "How long have you seen your most long-standing client?" This question will help you avoid the massage therapist that no one goes back to a second time.

9. Do you have references that I could call?

Ask for references' names and contact details and make sure you actually call or e-mail these people. Ideal references also have chronic pain issues.

Ask these referrals, "What do you like about this massage therapist?" "Have you ever been unusually sore afterwards?" and "Would you send your best friend to this person?"

Also ask the massage therapist, "Do you have a network of people who refer in and out to you?" A good massage therapist is well positioned in the community and continually works with doctors, physical therapists, psychologists, and dentists.

10. What are your rates? What is your cancellation policy?

Rates vary from as little as $30 per hour to more than $100. Find out in advance if your health insurance provider will pay for any portion of a therapeutic massage. If so, ask the massage therapist for a written receipt or form that you can submit. Inquire about possible discounts.

Also ask about the cancellation policy. Some massage therapists resent clients missing appointments without prior notification and may charge you for appointment no-shows. Finally, make sure the massage therapist's schedule and location are convenient to your needs.

❯ The Magic Question

Do you know where the eighteen fibromyalgia tender points are located?

If this massage therapist claims to know fibromyalgia, this question will prove it. Take a tender point/pain diagram with you to your appointment but show it to the massage therapist only *after* you've asked this question.

An alternative Magic Question for someone without prior knowledge of fibromyalgia or pain relief is, "Why did you want to become a massage therapist?" The best answers include sincerely passionate statements about "helping people."

YOUR 10 MOST EMBARRASSING MASSAGE QUESTIONS ANSWERED

Modesty may hinder your enjoyment and pain relief. The basic message is, "Don't worry about it." A reputable, experienced massage therapist has seen it all before. The following was adapted from About.com.

1. **Do I want a man or a woman massage therapist?**
   Consider this question before scheduling an appointment and don't hesitate to vocalize your preference.
2. **Do I take off my underwear?**
   Underwear is optional for a full body massage. Licensed massage therapists in North

America are required to make sure you are covered with a sheet or towel and use draping techniques on body parts not being massaged.

3. **Will the massage therapist watch me undress?**

   North American practitioners will leave the room and knock before reentering and after you've gotten under the sheet.

4. **What if the massage therapist touches my private parts?**

   A licensed massage therapist will not touch your genitals or nipples.

5. **What if I don't want the massage therapist to see a part of my body I'm self-conscious about?**

   If you worry about your weight, excessive body hair, unsightly feet, or scars, ask the massage therapist to avoid this area or request the massage through your clothing. Just remember the massage therapist has probably already seen much worse than you and you may hamper the therapeutic benefits of a full-body massage.

6. **What if I drool or fart during the massage?**

   Ask for a tissue, excuse yourself, laugh, or just ignore it. It happens all the time.

7. **What if I get turned on during the massage?**

   Some men hesitate to get a massage because they worry about having an erection. It does happen occasionally during a nonsexual, therapeutic massage. A professional therapist will ignore it. Or you can keep your underwear on and relax.

8. **Do I talk to the massage therapist during the session?**

   Chit-chat is optional. Your only job is to relax. Massage therapists don't expect you to talk. But be sure to speak up if you are in pain, uncomfortable, or have questions.

9. **What if I don't like the massage therapist's technique?**

   It's important that you communicate openly at that moment, especially if you are in pain. Don't just lie there and "take it." M. K. Brennan says, "For some clients, even the lightest touch can be too much."

10. **Do I tip the massage therapist?**

    There are no set rules but a 15 to 20 percent tip is considered standard if you are pleased with the services or for a massage in a hotel or spa. Some private practitioners don't expect or accept tips. Ask if you are unsure.

CONCLUSION

A good massage with gentle, knowing hands can feel heaven sent. Take the time to do your homework well when looking for a great massage therapist by asking Best Questions in advance.

You'll be less likely to feel shy, get hurt, or waste your money. If in doubt, check with your doctor beforehand.

THE 10 BEST RESOURCES

American Massage Therapy Association. "AMTA's Find a Massage Therapist." www.amtamassage.org/findamassage/locator.aspx.

American Massage Therapy Association. "Consumer Guide." www.amtamassage.org/consumers.html.

American Massage Therapy Association. "State Boards Administering Massage Practice Laws." www.amtamassage.org/pdf/2006_StateLaws.pdf.

Fibromyalgia-Symptoms.org. "Massage Therapy." www.fibromyalgia-symptoms.org/fibromyalgia_massage.html.

Mayo Clinic. "Massage." www.mayoclinic.com/health/massage/SA00082.

MedicineNet. "Massage Therapy." www.medicinenet.com/massage_therapy/article.htm.

National Center for Complementary and Alternative Medicine. "Massage Therapy as CAM." http://nccam.nih.gov/health/massage.

National Certification Board for Therapeutic Massage & Bodywork. "State Boards & Legislators." www.ncbtmb.org/legislators.php.

National Fibromyalgia Association. "Massage for Fibromyalgia: A Therapist's Point of View." www.fmaware.org/site/News2?page=News Article&id=6159.

ProHealth.com. "Hospitals Getting a Grip: Massage Therapy Finds Place in Patient Care for FM and More." www.prohealth.com/library/showarticle.cfm?id=6151&t=CFIDS_FM.

CHAPTER 13: THE 10 BEST QUESTIONS

For Choosing a Top Acupuncturist

The body never lies.

—Martha Graham

Acupuncture is defined as a technique of inserting thin needles through the skin at specific points on the body to control pain and other symptoms. As an alternative therapy to promote natural healing, acupuncture is earning a growing respect from the traditional medical community.

A 2005 Mayo Clinic study concluded that acupuncture significantly improves fibromyalgia symptoms, especially pain, anxiety, and fatigue. Dr. Brent A. Bauer, the director of the Complementary and Integrative Medicine Program at the Mayo Clinic, comments, "I recommend acupuncture for many of the patients who are referred to me and who have fibromyalgia. When I share this with their referring physicians, they are often at first surprised. But when I tell them of the research experience here at Mayo using acupuncture for fibromyalgia symptom treatment, they are quick to adopt it."

However tempting acupuncture may sound, you may hesitate due to fear of the unknown. Get your doctor's blessing first, and then ask the following Best Questions to find a well-qualified acupuncturist near you.

THE QUESTION DOCTOR SAYS:

Before you begin your search, find out if your insurance company covers acupuncture for fibromyalgia symptoms. Ask your insurance company these questions:

> Is this kind of treatment covered in my health-care plan?

> Are there any limits or requirements (like a restriction on the number of visits or the total amount allowed for payments)?

> Can I chose my own acupuncturist or do I have to see someone in your network?

> Do I need a referral from my doctor?

>>> THE 10 BEST QUESTIONS
For Choosing a Top Acupuncturist

1. Do you hold a current license to practice acupuncture and oriental medicine in this state?

Forty-eight states (excluding Wyoming and North Dakota) regulate acupuncture through reviews by state licensing boards. The National Certification Commission for Acupuncture and Oriental Medicine (NCCAOM) protects the public by ensuring licensed acupuncturists have the proper credentials. See their Web site at www.nccaom.org, which includes acupuncturists under disciplinary review.

Dr. Tess Hahn, the NCCAOM's current Chair of the Board of Commissioners and an Idaho-based professional acupuncturist says, "Utilize your state license board to make sure this acupuncturist has a current, active standing license to practice acupuncture."

Consumers should beware of medical professionals who do acupuncture as a sideline service but lack this license. The reason is that most medical doctors, naturopaths, and chiropractors who offer acupuncture have taken only 200–300 hours of training.

Dr. Tess Hahn advises, "Compare this requirement to the typical 3000–4000 hours of training that a licensed acupuncturist must complete. In most states, the requirements of acupuncture training for a non-M.D. acupuncturist are actually far greater than that of an M.D. practitioner. People may incorrectly assume that an M.D. would be better or more qualified to render treatment using acupuncture."

Another concern is that M.D.s are not required to use disposable needles as mandated for licensed acupuncturists. Some medical professionals truly love acupuncture, but many more use it primarily as a profitable sideline.

2. Are you an NCCAOM-certified acupuncturist?

The gold standard for acupuncturists is NCCAOM Diplomate status. Look for these initials after the person's name: OMD (Doctorate in Oriental Medicine), L.Ac. (Licensed Acupuncturist), or other abbreviations as explained at NCCAOM's Web site: www.nccaom.org/diplomates/index.html.

The "Dipl. Ac. (NCCAOM)" designation indicates this acupuncturist has been trained at a properly accredited facility and has passed the rigorous NCCAOM competency examination. There are about fifty-five accredited schools, but many more that are not. Diplomates are expected to take continuing education courses and must renew their certification every four years.

3. What has been your experience with treating people with fibromyalgia?

The best answer includes specifics such as the number of cases or how many treatments given per fibromyalgia patient. If you have limited choices for acupuncturists, ask about this person's experience in treating chronic pain.

Two excellent follow-up questions to ask are, "How does your technique for treating fibromyalgia patients differ from your technique for treating healthy individuals?" and "What results have you achieved with your fibromyalgia/chronic pain patients?" The most experienced acupuncturists will not hesitate to supply detailed, informative answers.

4. Besides acupuncture, which other modalities of oriental medicine do you use in cases such as mine?

There are five branches of oriental medicine, with acupuncture being just one of the branches. The other branches are Chinese medical/herbal therapy, Asian bodywork therapy, exercise and **qigong therapy** (energy flow techniques like tai chi), and dietary and lifestyle therapy.

As Dr. Tess Hahn explains, "When I treat patients with fibromyalgia, I don't just do acupuncture. I use a combined approach. For instance, I often prescribe medicinal herbs in liquid or tablet form. There are about four thousand Chinese herbs combined into several hundred formulas which have been used for twenty-five hundred years. It's a big body of knowledge, so you want someone who really knows which one to use for which person."

5. Please tell me about your initial examination.

A good sign is an actively involved acupuncturist asking you lots of questions during a comprehensive initial examination. She will be determining exactly where and how the pain shows up in your body.

This initial exam helps the acupuncturist focus on stimulating the right points on you for pain relief and recovery. Examples of typical exam questions include details about your sleeping patterns, appetite, and elimination.

6. What makes acupuncture so important to you that you chose to become a professional acupuncturist?

Answers will vary. You may hear the acupuncturist's personal story about how he conquered his own health challenges.

Also listen for clues into how focused this acupuncturist is on improving your quality of life and what values are important to him about his chosen career.

7. What is your greatest strength or special interest as an acupuncturist?

As in other health professions, most practitioners don't treat all types of cases all the time. For example, Dr. Tess Hahn says, "I know I'm not strong in pediatrics, but I treat a lot of fibromyalgia patients because I enjoy helping them. My colleagues send me their pain patients when they don't get results." That's an ideal response.

8. How do most of your patients find you?

Look for an acupuncturist who is so successful that he can rely exclusively on word-of-mouth referrals for new business. While there's nothing wrong with advertising, especially for new practitioners, the ones who operate by referrals alone know they have to work extra hard to maintain their good reputations.

Ask about a waiting list, which can be an initial irritant but ultimately is a good sign. It's the same principle as a long line of people waiting to get into a popular restaurant.

9. Do I fill out my own insurance forms or does your office do that?

Ninety-five percent of professional acupuncturists are self-employed. Therefore, your acupuncturist probably doesn't have the staff or resources to submit insurance claims on your behalf.

Ask if this acupuncturist provides a receipt called a "super bill." This is a standard form used to report treatments to insurance providers.

10. Are you interested in treating me? Why?

Dr. Tess Hahn suggested these questions along with, "What do you think you can do to improve my life?" and "Are you excited about doing that?" It only makes sense that you want someone who really cares and is passionate about her ability to help you.

> The Magic Question

Do you know where the eighteen fibromyalgia tender points are located?

If this acupuncturist claims to know about fibromyalgia and trigger points, here's a little quiz for her. There's no reason to be confrontational about how you ask this question.

If the answer is no, but you like this person anyway, you may want to educate her about fibromyalgia. Take a tender point diagram with you or use your body to explain. But chances are a well-qualified practitioner knows way more than you do.

CONCLUSION

Acupuncture helps your body find the potential to heal itself. This process requires a great deal of knowledge and the skillful hands of an experienced and licensed acupuncturist.

As Dr. Tess Hahn concludes, "There is 'cookbook acupuncture' for very simple things, and then there's true Oriental medicine as acupuncture techniques are applied specifically for an individual's health pattern. The distinction between these two is really key and lies in the diagnosis. A correct initial assessment of what's going on with that person is very important. You want a practitioner who has a very detailed understanding of the patterns of disharmony in the body and treats every patient differently."

THE 10 BEST RESOURCES

AcuFinder.com. "Search Acupuncturists." www.acufinder.com.

American Association of Acupuncture & Oriental Medicine. "Consumer Guide." www.aaaomonline.org/default.asp?pagenumber=10.

American Organization for Bodywork Therapies of Asia. "AOBTA Directory." www.aobta.org/aobta-directory.html?sobi2Task=search.

Council of Colleges of Acupuncture and Oriental Medicine. "Know Your Acupuncturist." www.ccaom.org/downloads/KnowYourAcupuncturist.pdf.

Mayo Clinic. "Acupuncture: Can It Help?" www.mayoclinic.com/health/acupuncture/SA00086.

Mayo Clinic. "Acupuncture Relieves Symptoms of Fibromyalgia, Mayo Clinic Study Finds." www.mayoclinic.org/news2006-rst/3495.html.

MedicineNet. "Acupuncture." www.medicinenet.com/acupuncture/article.htm.

National Center for Complementary and Alternative Medicine. "Introduction to Acupuncture." http://nccam.nih.gov/health/acupuncture.

National Fibromyalgia Association. "Acupuncture." www.fmaware.org/site/PageServer?pagename=topics_acupuncture.

WebMD. "Study: Acupuncture Helps Fibromyalgia." www.webmd.com/fibromyalgia/news/20050824/study-acupuncture-helps-fibromyalgia.

PART III:

Making Healthy Lifestyle Changes

Use the Best Questions in this section to proactively improve your health habits. For example, many people with fibromyalgia want to find new ways to incorporate exercise and a better diet into their lives, but just don't know how to get started. You can't undo a lifetime of eating Big Macs, smoking, and inactivity overnight, but asking yourself the right questions is a great start.

If you are among the large group of people with fibromyalgia who suffer from sleep disturbances, look at chapter 14 for the Best Questions and tips on getting good sleep. Be kind to yourself and really honest in your self-assessment of your stress in chapter 15, and losing weight and eating healthier in chapter 16.

Most people, even the healthiest ones, don't get enough exercise. Oregon Health & Science University's fibromyalgia expert, Dr. Kim Dupree Jones, offers straight-talking advice for people with fibromyalgia, "Get more exercise into your life." A really good start is finding a great gym or fitness club (chapter 17) and getting guidance from a top personal fitness trainer (chapter 18). Making exercise a lifelong healthy habit will be easier.

It's worth it. Even if you've had great doctors, found the right fibromyalgia medications and therapies, and your symptoms are in remission, nothing trumps a healthy lifestyle in your battle for good health.

CHAPTER 14: THE 10 BEST QUESTIONS
To Get a Good Night's Sleep

The worst thing in the world is to try to sleep and not to.
—F. Scott Fitzgerald

The National Sleep Foundation estimates that 60 percent of adults have trouble sleeping at least a few nights a week. According to a 2004 *New York Times* interview with Dr. Meir H. Kryger, a former president of the American Academy of Sleep Medicine, an estimated 40–80 million people in the United States suffer from **insomnia,** a sleep disorder defined as the inability to fall or stay asleep when you want to, and **sleep deprivation,** the general lack of necessary sleep that is often self-induced to cram more activities into the day.

An estimated 80 percent of people with fibromyalgia have sleeping disorders, including chronic insomnia, **restless legs syndrome,** and **periodic limb movement disorder** (periodic nighttime movements). Dr. Harvey Moldofsky, a professor emeritus at the University of Toronto and a fibromyalgia research pioneer, discovered that people with fibromyalgia demonstrate abnormal brain activity and other sleep abnormalities.

Dr. Charles R. Cantor, a sleep medicine expert and the medical director of the Penn Sleep Centers of the University of Pennsylvania, explains, "Chronic pain and sleep difficulties are mutually reinforcing in a negative way. When you have a lot of pain it interferes with your sleep. When you have poor quality sleep, it makes your pain worse. It's a vicious cycle. The good news is that you can treat both pain and sleep disturbances. But if you treat only one of them, you aren't going to do as well."

Several fibromyalgia sufferers share their sleep stories. Dot Gerecke of Horsham, Australia describes her sleeping habits as "way off beat." Singer/songwriter Rosie Hamlin recalls, "I used to have restless legs syndrome all over my body. My muscles kept jumping and twitching at night." Linda Pütz, a Maryland-based career coach, recommends talking with a cognitive behavioral sleep therapist. She says, "Finally, here was someone that was actually trained to talk with me about **sleep hygiene** (sleep habits and environmental factors)."

If you have trouble getting a good night's sleep, ask yourself these Best Questions as a checklist to assess what simple changes in your own sleep hygiene may help you.

>>> THE 10 BEST QUESTIONS
To Get a Good Night's Sleep

1. How sleepy am I during the day?

Many people get sleepy in the afternoon. But if you are sleepy all the time or tend to fall asleep throughout the day, you may not be getting enough quality sleep.

Daytime sleepiness is a good clue about how effective your sleep is. Many people who think they are sleeping poorly actually function well during the day and may not have to worry about their sleep as much as they think they do.

Sleep expert Dr. Charles R. Cantor recommends that you take a quick, useful quiz called the Epworth Sleepiness Scale to determine how likely you are to fall asleep in various situations. Find it along with a short analysis at http://en.wikipedia.org/wiki/Epworth_Sleepiness_Scale. If you have an abnormal Epworth score, tell your doctor about it.

Sleep experts believe that naps can disturb nighttime sleep

patterns. A 2008 study published in the journal *Sleep* found that napping habits were tied to higher levels of nighttime sleep fragmentation, respiratory problems, and pain in older people. Avoid daytime napping if possible, or limit your naps to fewer than forty-five minutes before three o'clock p.m.

2. How sleepy am I at bedtime?

Sleep experts advise you shouldn't go to bed unless you are sleepy. Try to build your bedtime schedule around a time that's your natural sleep time. Read a book or listen to soft music to help you relax.

If you aren't asleep in twenty minutes, get out of bed, go to another room, and do something relaxing or boring (reading, etc.). Once you feel sleepy again, go back to bed. Avoid the television or computer because they can over-stimulate you. Don't watch the clock either because it can increase your anxiety about not being able to sleep.

3. Am I going to bed and getting up at approximately the same time every day?

Decide on a bedtime and an awakening time and stick to them, including weekends and holidays. You want your body used to being asleep at certain, relatively fixed times. Even if you aren't working or are retired, this habit is essential to good sleeping hygiene.

4. Do I have bedtime "rituals" that help me relax before bedtime?

It's easier to fall asleep if you establish and stick to "rituals" like taking a warm, relaxing bath before bed and brushing your teeth. This keeps your inner clock running smoothly. Sleep experts also advise that you keep a regular schedule for your meals, medications, chores, and other daily activities.

5. Am I using stimulants that could disturb my sleep?

Many people falsely believe alcohol aids relaxation when in fact it is a stimulant and should be avoided in the evening. Do not have beer, wine, or any other alcohol within six hours of your bedtime.

Other stimulants to skip during afternoon and evening hours include caffeine (coffee, tea, chocolate, and many sodas), nicotine, and sugary or spicy foods. For best results, don't go to bed hungry, but don't sleep on a full stomach either. In general, exercise will help you sleep, but avoid vigorous exercise near bedtime.

6. Am I using my bedroom for activities other than sleeping or sex?

One of the worst things you can do for your sleeping problems is to use your bedroom for other activities. Sleep experts say you shouldn't watch television, use your computer, eat, write, talk on the phone, or anything else in bed or in your bedroom.

When you use your bedroom for other activities, merely walking into your bedroom causes your brain to literally wake up because it automatically associates being in that room with being mentally alert. Moving your television or computer out of your bedroom can have a surprisingly positive effect on your sleep.

However, for many people with fibromyalgia this is an acknowledged challenge. Dr. Kim Dupree Jones, a fibromyalgia expert at the Oregon Health & Science University, says, "Some people with severe fibromyalgia almost live in their beds, which is a real problem. If so, invest in a very comfortable chair for a room that's not your bedroom. Then when you are in your bedroom, your body can associate your bed with going to sleep."

7. Is my sleeping environment as comfortable as possible?

You may not have considered your obvious sleeping needs, like comfortable bedding, a good pillow, and eliminating distractions.

Make sure there is very little noise or light when you are sleeping, which can be especially troublesome for people with fibromyalgia. Find a comfortable sleeping position. Ask others not to disturb you or sleep alone.

Think of your bedroom as your cave—dark, quiet, and a little cool. No wonder bats and bears who sleep in dark caves are such champion snoozers!

8. How are my emotions, stress, and depression contributing to my sleeping problems?

Your bed is a place to rest, not a place to worry. One of the big causes of insomnia is stress.

As Dr. Charles R. Cantor explains, "Psychological factors play into both pain and poor sleep. People who have chronic pain get frustrated and discouraged, and these emotions tend to undermine good sleep and make insomnia worse. This creates further anxiety about sleep and you develop a 'performance anxiety.' Then your responses to pain and to poor sleep reinforce each other."

Try to avoid getting too fixated and overreacting to your sleep problems. For some people, just seeing their bed fills them with despair. If you are at this point, talk to your doctor or seek specialized help from a sleep medicine expert, neurologist, or psychologist. Chapters 2 through 5 will help you find a good sleep doctor.

9. What medications might help me to sleep better? Could any of my current medications be causing my insomnia? What are my options?

"Your doctor will know more about the various medications than you do, but if he doesn't know you are having trouble sleeping, he won't be able to connect the dots and help you," says Dr. Charles R. Cantor. "If you have expectations, beliefs, or fears about sleeping pills, you need to have a frank discussion with your doctor."

Some sleeping pills can also help chronic pain. See more in chapter 8.

Other fibromyalgia drugs can cause or aggravate sleeping disturbances, such as an antidepressant that sometimes causes restless legs syndrome. Another example is beta blockers prescribed for heart conditions that also affect sleep quality.

An alternative to medications is a **cognitive behavioral therapy** that emphasizes good sleep hygiene education. See the American Academy of Sleep Medicine's Web site (www.aasmnet.org/BSMSpecialists.aspx) for a certified sleep specialist near you or ask your doctor for a referral.

10. What does my bed partner tell me about my sleeping habits?

Dr. Charles R. Cantor suggested that you may not have considered your bed partner as a source of information on sleep problems that you need to discuss with your doctor. Your bed partner can tell you if you snore or have unusual sleep behaviors such as restlessness or talking in your sleep.

Of particular concern is to ask your bed partner if you snore while sleeping. Excessive snoring, especially if it's punctuated with periods of silence or nonbreathing, may indicate **sleep apnea**. Sleep apnea is the condition in which sleep is repeatedly disrupted due to disturbed breathing patterns. It often results in foggy-headed days, sleep deprivation, and contributes to hypertension and heart disease. Being obese increases the odds for having this condition. Experts warn that the combination of poor sleep, hypertension, and obesity is potentially deadly.

ASK YOUR DOCTOR: DO I NEED A SLEEP STUDY?

It's important to talk with your doctor about your sleeping difficulties. He may suggest a **sleep study** to evaluate and analyze the quality of your sleep. Fibromyalgia expert Dr. Patrick Wood advises, "When sleep apnea contributes to fibromyalgia, a sleep study is highly recommended."

Dr. Charles R. Cantor agrees but with this caveat, "If you have trouble falling asleep, a sleep study may not help much because you just lie awake all night trying to get to sleep. But if your problem is staying asleep, a sleep study can help you understand what's disturbing your sleep."

〉The Magic Question

Could I have another sleep disorder independent of fibromyalgia?

Dr. Kim Dupree Jones says, "Sleep is so key in fibromyalgia. Treating sleep problems is so important."

It is, but patients and doctors sometimes get so focused on treating the fibromyalgia-induced sleeping problems that they miss other warning signs. Dr. Charles R. Cantor explains, "It's important that you and your doctor don't just assume that your sleeping problems are related to your fibromyalgia. You may have symptoms that will lead your doctor to suspect something else is going on, like sleep apnea. People can fall through the cracks this way."

Ask both yourself and your doctor this Magic Question.

CONCLUSION

Even though sleep disruptions are very common among fibromyalgia patients, many don't realize that they can take proactive measures to improve their odds of getting a good night's sleep. It's empowering to realize some sleeping issues are within your control to change.

Many sleep deprived people with fibromyalgia suffer in silence, thinking that their sleeping problems aren't worth discussing with their doctors or they are too embarrassed to bring them up. The sleep experts advise both patients and physicians to move beyond this attitude.

Sleep disorders are not your cross to bear, and are treatable with medications and behavioral changes. As Dr. Charles R. Cantor concludes, "It's important to tell your doctor what your sleep schedule is, how well you think you are sleeping, and what your perceived sleeping difficulties are."

Sweet dreams. Zzzzzzzzzzzzzzzzz.

THE 10 BEST RESOURCES

American Academy of Family Physicians. "Insomnia: How to Get a Good Night's Sleep." http://familydoctor.org/online/famdocen/home/articles/110.html.

American Academy of Sleep Medicine. "SleepEducation.com's Home Page." www.sleepeducation.com/index.aspx.

Cleveland Clinic. "Choosing a Doctor and Finding a Sleep Center." http://my.clevelandclinic.org/disorders/Sleep_Disorders/hic_Choosing_a_Doctor_and_Finding_a_Sleep_Center.aspx.

Mayo Clinic. "Sleep Center." www.mayoclinic.com/health/sleep/SL99999.

MedlinePlus. "Sleep Disorders." www.nlm.nih.gov/medlineplus/sleepdisorders.html.

National Sleep Foundation. "A to zzzzs." www.sleepfoundation.org/site/c.huIXKjM0IxF/b.2462635/apps/nl/co ntent3.asp?content_id={ADDFC78C-7DE8-4823-B71D-702B928CAF3A}&notoc=1.

SleepCenters.org. "Locate a Sleep Center by State." www.sleepcenters.org/index.aspx.

SleepEducation. "Sleep Hygiene." www.sleepeducation.com/Hygiene.aspx.

SleepEducation. "Sleepiness Scale." www.sleepeducation.com/SleepScale.aspx.

WebMD. "Find a Sleep Specialist." www.webmd.com/sleep-disorders/sleep-specialists.

CHAPTER 15: THE 10 BEST QUESTIONS

To Tame Your Stress

> Stress is an ignorant state. It believes that everything is an emergency.
>
> —Natalie Goldberg, author

There is mounting evidence that stress harms your health as much as a bad diet or lack of exercise. But because most doctors are extremely busy, and are ironically cramming more and more patient appointments into their already crowded calendars, very few have the time to sit and have a long, leisurely physician-patient chat about your stress levels. Your doctor may have the best intentions, but realistically she can't do much about the fact that you were laid off from your job last year or that your husband left you last week.

So it's up to you to slow down, take an honest look at what's causing your stress, and consider how much your stress and emotional state may be affecting your pain levels. The American Institute of Stress says that patients and doctors often overlook stress management as a health issue and a treatment option.

Martha Beck, well-known fibromyalgia patient, life coach, and bestselling author, says, "After my diagnosis, I changed my whole life so I would have very little stress in it. I work hard but it's joyful. There's very little that I do in my profession that I don't absolutely love."

A 2007 survey by the National Fibromyalgia Association concluded that at least 40 percent of people with fibromyalgia suffer from stress and anxiety. Some researchers think that when stress continues without relief, your body triggers physical reactions that can lead to fibromyalgia.

Reducing stress as a fibromyalgia remedy is probably one of the easiest and safest treatments possible. You can avoid drugs' side effects, pay little or nothing, and enjoy broader health benefits as well.

Taking the time to slow down and savor the small moments is a life skill that is difficult for most people, but it pays great rewards. Our busy lives keep us moving so fast that we often miss out on the things that are truly important. Each of us has experienced moments of peace, depth, and meaning. But it's tough to make daily relaxation as normal as brushing your teeth.

The first step in de-stressing your life is an honest self-assessment of what's causing your stress. Download all of your free-floating brain and artery-clogging gotta-do's for a few minutes while you ask yourself the following Best Questions.

THE QUESTION DOCTOR SAYS:

Consider seeing a professional counselor or therapist if your stress is out of control or you're having trouble understanding its causes and solutions. To find a reputable therapist, adjust the Best Questions in chapters 2, 3, and 4 and start asking.

>>>THE 10 BEST QUESTIONS
To Tame Your Stress

1. When is the last time I felt really relaxed?
Think back. Feel your nerves relax and your throat unclench. What were you doing? Where were you? Why were you relaxed? What relaxes you the most?

Capture your relaxed moments and examine them. What do they have in common? What small piece of this relaxed freedom can you re-create on a daily basis?

This reflection can also be examined from the perspective of the work done by Dr. Herbert Benson, a pioneer in mind-body connections and author of the classic book *The Relaxation Response*. He says, "The Relaxation Response is the biological opposite of the fight-or-flight response. It comes about when you break your train of everyday thoughts by choosing a word to focus on. This word should be repetitive and have meaning, like *love, peace,* or a *prayer*.

2. Why am I stressed? What major life changes have I had to deal with within the last year?

From the death of a spouse or a divorce to getting a speeding ticket, stressful events take their toll on our health and well-being. The practical Life Events Questionnaire (also called the Holmes and Rahe Stress Scale) is a list of forty-one stressful life events that can contribute to illness. You can easily take this highly respected and well validated test yourself to assess your risk of stress-induced illness. See http://en.wikipedia.org/wiki/Holmes_and_Rahe_stress_scale.

3. How much is worry or stress affecting my sleep?

Lost sleep robs us of the ability to restore ourselves physically, mentally, and emotionally. Previous studies have found links between poor sleep and significant metabolic and endocrine changes that mimic the aging process, high levels of **cortisol** (the body's stress hormone), and weight gain. See more in chapter 14.

4. Has anyone close to me told me they were worried about my stress level?

Does this sound familiar? Friends and family have pleaded with you, asking for nothing more than a simple phone call. Please, they ask, let me know you're okay.

Or perhaps you've been asked by an old friend, "Are you okay? You don't look so good. Are you still working all that overtime?"

5. If I'm really honest with myself, how much do I think excessive stress contributes to my fibromyalgia?

No one knows the exact correlation yet and fibromyalgia is still viewed by many as a "mysterious" disease, but some experts suggest that chronic stress may aggravate the body's immune system and somehow be related to chronic pain.

For some people with fibromyalgia, stress levels are further heightened because they get so little support or sympathy about their pain from the other people in their lives. This pain-stress cycle then becomes a vicious circle.

6. How much does my job contribute to my stress?

Move over, road rage. Here comes desk rage. And it's getting worse. Anger in the workplace stemming from grumpy coworkers and insulting supervisors in addition to intense feelings of frustration, fear, and being overwhelmed, is growing.

The American Institute of Stress states that job stress is by far the leading cause of stress for American adults. Eighty percent of workers feel stressed on the job with nearly half saying they need help. A full 25 percent of American workers view their jobs as the number one stressor in their lives.

Workplace stress consultant Anna Maravelas says, "Be especially careful not to conclude that you're trapped at work. Telling ourselves we have no options causes stress to skyrocket. If your best friend was describing your work situation to you, what advice would you give him or her?"

Management consultant Sharon Jordan-Evans also offers advice. She says, "As people go into that workplace quandary, 'Should I stay or should I go?' they should first try to find out what's missing and what's wrong in their current job."

7. When I'm stressed, what do I do about it? How well do I recognize stress in myself?

It's important to identify the sources of stress in your life so that you can try to avoid or reduce them. External sources of stress include work pressures, family relationships, and financial worries.

There is also self-generated stress in people with type A behavior, which is characterized by a fiercely competitive spirit and unrealistic self-imposed expectations. Type A behavior can kill. It is a significant risk factor for coronary heart disease as well.

8. If I wasn't feeling stressed, what would be different?

This question is borrowed from the thinking of **solution focused brief therapists.** They believe that if people can identify the things they wish they could change in their lives, they are capable of constructing a "preferred future" for themselves. Go to www .sfbta.org.

You can work on developing your own preferred future by asking yourself (or working with a therapist) to construct "what if" questions, like, "What if I woke up tomorrow and a miracle happened that took away all the pain and stress in my life?" "What if I loved my job?" Some people find novel solutions with this innovative approach that examines the gap between current reality and their ideal state.

9. Do I set standards or expectations for myself that are too high to really achieve?

Many stressed-out people are perfectionists, always striving to get it all right, keep all the balls in the air, and make Superman or Superwoman look like a rookie. Chronic stress can result from a lifelong history of getting straight As in school, winning key promotions, and expecting your kids to be on the honor roll as well as world-class soccer players.

You must consciously break this cycle by seeking stress-reduction techniques, finding more pleasure in smaller sandboxes, and demanding less of yourself and your loved ones. So what if your garden has weeds or your son flunked band class?

10. Who and what can help me the most to reduce the stress in my life?

Stress management gurus advise tackling stress at its root causes. The healthy lifestyle changes you are making (more exercise, healthy diet, etc.) will also tame your stress.

Finding good emotional support can make a huge difference. Consider a fibromyalgia support group or reconnecting with the people who make you happiest. Find ways to build in more "time-outs" during your everyday life, including quick power naps or meditative moments.

And consider the wisdom of business guru Stephen Covey when he says, "Begin with the end in mind." Charlie Chaplin also got it right when he said, "Nothing is permanent in this wicked world, not even our troubles."

❯ The Magic Question

What is my preferred antidote to stress? How destructive or constructive is it?

Another way of asking this question may be, "What is my favorite poison?" Although some people find smart solutions to stress, like physical activities, favorite hobbies, fun vacations, or playing with their kids, most of us also have destructive behavior patterns that we use as stress reducers.

Harvard University's cardiac specialist Dr. Daniel Forman comments, "Our ways of dealing with stress are often self-destructive, like overeating, smoking, or watching TV." Dr. Herbert Benson adds, "The intensity of a person's fight-or-flight response to stress is determined by that individual's interpretation of its meaning."

Ask yourself whether there is any substance or food that you would have trouble living without. You'll probably immediately consider cigarettes, alcohol, chocolate, bread, or coffee. These addictive stimulants and foods provide short-term energy boosts but can add to your long-term health problems and stress.

A good indication of the impact these substances or foods have on you is what happens when they are withdrawn. For example, many people get headaches when their bodies are deprived of caffeine.

However, such symptoms are usually followed by a feeling of lightness and increased energy as the body is freed from the burden of coping with the toxins created by these substances. Just ask anyone who has successfully quit smoking.

DO I HAVE POSTTRAUMATIC STRESS?

You may be a war veteran and suffer from **posttraumatic stress** (characterized by intense fear, helplessness, or horror after a terrifying event; also called the **Gulf War Syndrome**). Several studies have linked combat-related posttraumatic stress with the pain characteristic of fibromyalgia. One study concluded that almost half of the study's posttraumatic sufferers also met the criteria for a fibromyalgia diagnosis. See more in chapter 7, Best Question 4.

CONCLUSION

Stress is a common medical condition that is largely undiagnosed and untreated in millions of people. Medical research continues to reveal irrefutable connections between both the powers of stress and relaxation on our health. Just as stress has a chronic negative effect, regular relaxation has been shown to repair the damage caused by our response to stress.

Live to be one hundred years old. Relax into wellness.

THE 10 BEST RESOURCES

American Institute of Stress. "Topics of Interest." www.stress.org/topic-interest.htm?AIS=9f071b015d36caa499d75130bbaf19b3.

American Psychiatric Association. "Mental Health Resources." www.psych.org/Resources/MentalHealthResources.aspx.

Benson, Herbert. *The Relaxation Response*. New York: HarperCollins, 2000.

Kabat-Zinn, Jon. *Wherever You Go, There You Are: Mindfulness Meditation in Everyday Life,* 10th ed. New York: Hyperion, 2005.

Leider, Richard J. *The Power of Purpose: Creating Meaning in Your Life and Work*. San Francisco: Berrett-Koehler, 1997.

Maravelas, Anna. *How to Reduce Workplace Conflict and Stress: How Leaders and Their Employees Can Protect Their Sanity and Productivity from Tension and Turf Wars*. Franklin Lakes: NJ: Career Press, 2005.

National Fibromyalgia Association. "Stress." www.fmaware.org/site/PageServer?pagename=topics_stress.

University of Massachusetts Medical School. "Stress Reduction Program." www.umassmed.edu/Content.aspx?id=41254.

WebMD. "Posttraumatic Stress, Fibromyalgia Linked." www.webmd.com/news/20040610/posttraumatic-stress-fibromyalgia-linked.

Wikipedia. "Stress (biological)." http://en.wikipedia.org/wiki/Stress_%28medicine%29.

CHAPTER 16: THE 10 BEST QUESTIONS

To Lose Weight and Eat Well

> Life expectancy would grow by leaps and bounds if green
> vegetables smelled as good as bacon.
>
> —Doug Larson, British runner

There's a lot of truth to Andy Rooney's observation, "The biggest seller is cookbooks and the second is diet books—how not to eat what you've just learned how to cook."

Many people are confused. For example, top nutritional experts alternatively swear by a dizzying selection of olive oil, no oil, flax-seed oil, butter, margarine, and even lard as best choices. Everywhere we look we are bombarded by fad diets, pictures of skinny celebrities and six-pack-ab guys, cheap fast foods, and tons of tempting sweets. No wonder so many people are overweight or obese.

Your health challenges may be just the right wake-up call to finally take charge of your weight issues. There is no specific diet recommended for people with fibromyalgia, but many medical experts suspect there are important food connections and ones to avoid. Common cautions include stimulants, such as caffeine, alcohol, and chocolate, especially after midday for sleep problems. Try to also reduce additives and preservatives like MSG, salt, and the seasonings in soup, canned food, prepackaged goods, and fast foods, which can sensitize the central nervous system and drive pain.

The following Best Questions don't promise a miracle cure. But asking yourself these questions will help you understand your own eating behaviors and weaknesses, set more realistic long-term goals, and hopefully inspire you to maintain good weight and make healthy food choices during your entire lifetime. See chapter 6 for questions to ask your doctor about weight and diet management.

THE QUESTION DOCTOR SAYS:

Why is pie not the answer? It's because the word *desserts* is *stressed* spelled backward.

>>>THE 10 BEST QUESTIONS
To Lose Weight and Eat Well

1. What am I doing to control my portion sizes?

The Muppets' Miss Piggy once said, "Never eat more than you can lift." Portion size has a way of creeping up. We're influenced by a fast-food culture where more food equals better value. Time to get "unsupersized."

As a registered dietitian in Virginia, Peggy Jensen advises, "People spend a lot of time worrying about *what* they eat but not enough time thinking about *how much* they eat." If you eat half of your normal amounts, you can cut your calories by half without radically changing your favorite foods.

Here are some other time-tested tips. Eat just half a sandwich or half a bowl of ice cream. Chew slowly to let your stomach register it is full. Use smaller plates (salad-size) to downsize dinner portions. Buy snacks in smaller bags so you'll stop sooner. Keep second helpings out of sight. Remember the recommended serving sizes. For example, three ounces of meat is the size of a deck of cards, and a cup of potatoes looks like a tennis ball.

2. Am I willing to learn how to read and use the information on food labels?

Besides being a portion-control hawk, the most successful dieters are label fiends. Not knowing how to read the **Nutrition Facts** on labels is a big obstacle in achieving lifetime weight control. A clear explanation is offered by the U.S. Food and Drug Administration's Web site at www.cfsan.fda.gov/~dms/foodlab.html.

Also get in the habit of reading the list of ingredients. The list is in descending order by weight. By comparing cereal boxes, for example, you'll see that one brand has more whole wheat and fewer calories than another brand. Choose products with less sodium, corn fructose or corn syrup, saturated fats, and fewer long strings of unappealing chemicals.

As you get more experienced, you'll be able to spot food manufacturers' purposefully misleading statements (reduced-fat crackers with added salt) and confusing bird-size portions that deemphasize real calorie damage.

Cleveland Heart Clinic's preventive medicine consultant Dr. Caldwell B. Esselstyn advises, "Read the ingredients! And be careful not to get complacent."

3. Would my great-grandmother recognize this food?

Foods are transformed from their original state (like raw vegetables or fresh meat) into marketable food products called **processed foods.** Eating too many highly processed foods is a major cause of weight gain because they often contain refined sugars (think: diabetes epidemic), unhealthy additives, hidden salt and fat, and mystery ingredients (think: hot dogs). The goodness of natural food is usually lost in processing.

The University of Tennessee's nutrition expert Dr. Barbara

Clarke comments, "Our food has radically changed. Previously, fast food wasn't so available and grocery stores had limited choices."

Because processed foods are now so commonplace, you might have trouble identifying them. That's why you want to consider your great-grandmother's diet fifty or one hundred years ago. She knew lettuce but not processed vegetable chips and would have recognized frozen cherries but not cherry Kool-Aid.

If you can't channel your great-grandmother, try asking yourself, "Can I pick it, cut it, butcher it, or catch it?" or "Would a caveman recognize this food?" Both questions will help you sort out processed and natural food choices. Dr. Caldwell B. Esselstyn offers a simple vegetarian version of this Best Question: "Did my food have a face or a mother?"

4. What is my daily allowance for calories, fat grams, fiber grams, salt, and carbohydrates to maintain my weight? To lose weight?

The **Recommended Daily Allowance** (RDA) describes standard recommendations for a person's intake of essential nutrients to maintain a normal weight and a healthy body. These requirements vary widely based on gender, age, body size, and amount of physical activity.

Many people focus on daily calorie counts, which is a good start but ultimately insufficient for long-term nutritional health. See dietary guidance at this Web site: http://en.wikipedia.org/wiki/Recommended_daily_allowance.

To learn more about how to count your calories for weight loss, see the Calorie Control Council's Web site at www.caloriecontrol.org. If you have only a minimum knowledge about nutrition, ask your doctor or a dietitian for more guidance.

5. How frequently can I prepare more of my own food?

If you can cook, you win two big points in the diet war. Preparing at least some meals yourself can be invaluable in weight loss and management because you can control the quality of the ingredients. Dr. Barbara Clarke comments, "It's very important to have cooking skills to manage your diet in a simple, healthful, and controllable way."

Peggy Jensen agrees: "The biggest obstacle is a mind-set that I don't have time for this. It's not about preparing foods from scratch but preparing what you eat. When you get into it, you realize it doesn't take more time than the junky stuff."

Cooking can be tough for some people with fibromyalgia. Oregon fibromyalgia expert Dr. Kim Dupree Jones advises, "Fatigue is a huge problem with fibromyalgia, so use already cut-up fruits and vegetables to save your time and energy. That way, when you are already exhausted, you won't reach for fast food, but will eat more sensibly."

6. Who and what can help me achieve my diet and nutrition goals?

Recruit someone more objective about your weight and more knowledgeable about food choices to help you.

Dr. Barbara Clarke says, "If someone is trying to change their diet for medical reasons, they really need to sit down with a registered dietitian and plot out where they are and what can they reasonably change in small steps. We are talking about changing habits that people have had for a long, long time, but we put too much burden on the individual." Likewise, Peggy Jensen suggests, "You can buy shark cartilage on the Web, but a dietitian is going to tell you accurate information and support you."

Experts advise that record keeping is one of the most successful techniques for losing weight. Keep a food diary of everything you eat, its portion size, feelings associated with eating, and calorie count. You'll see patterns emerge that can identify your triggers for overeating. There are many online versions, or try this Web site: http://familydoctor.org/online/famdocen/home/healthy/food/general-nutrition/299.html.

7. Which foods am I willing to give up a few times a week? Which foods would I miss the most?

Without qualifying for full-time martyrdom, consider what bad foods are the easiest to give up, then the second easiest to give up, and so on. Taking your lifestyle changes in small steps will help big time with long-term victory.

Peggy Jensen also suggests asking yourself if you are willing to give up meat a few times a week. This may gradually help you adopt a more plant-based diet.

At the same time, don't forsake your favorite foods forever. Even strict dietitians agree this can be a recipe for a diet disaster. Your intense longing for a favorite food may result in a bingeing session later.

8. What are my smartest choices when I'm dining out?

In advance, check online menus for healthy selections. Ask for a take-out container for oversized restaurant portions or order from the children's menu. Resist upsized offers at fast-food restaurants (the dollar meal deal, etc.), and skip all-you-can-eat buffets.

Instead of choosing the tastiest menu item, retrain yourself to ask, "What is the healthiest thing I can order from this menu?" This wonderful Best Question can rescue you from many diet-sabotaging temptations.

Another consideration is that you may need to be prepared to eat differently from others in a social situation, such as dining at a friend's home. Gently insist that you don't need an overflowing plate or pass on dessert.

9. What is my snack strategy?

Peggy Jensen advises, "When you are hungry, all bets are off. Carry your own healthy snack foods, like nuts or fruit, with you so you won't eat junk food when you are tired or stressed out. When you are hungry, you are mad at the world."

Other smart snack strategies include choosing quality over quantity (a handful of nuts versus a big bag of chips), keeping variety in your snacks (like seasonal fruits, whole-grain crackers, or baby carrots), watching portion sizes, and satisfying cravings with better choices, like yogurt instead of candy or granola bars. Also be careful not to slip up after dinner, a prime time to gain weight because you are probably less active.

10. Is my diet plan one that I can stick with long term?

This diet has to really be your thing, not boring tofu or impossible meals to fix especially during fibromyalgia flare-ups and when you are exhausted. To make your diet plan really work, you first need to internalize this diet—make it work for *you*. Keep in mind that you are probably less active and thus burning fewer calories when you don't feel well or can't exercise.

Even if you cook for others, don't cook, or eat out frequently, practicing good nutrition every day is a commitment to yourself. It may take you a few weeks, months, or even years to really get and stay slim.

Work with your doctor or a dietitian to establish short- and long-term goals that are achievable, not just another source of stress for things you haven't done yet. Keep asking yourself Peggy Jensen's question, "What can I eat that is good for me and that I really like?"

❭ The Magic Question

Am I hungry enough to eat an apple?

Many people have been misusing food for so long they are out of touch with their body's true "I'm hungry, feed me" signals. Eating out of habit or to alleviate pain or difficult emotions, such as stress, depression, or fatigue, is very, very common.

One way to get back in touch with your body's true food needs is to choose a food that you like okay, like apples, but don't dream about, like brownies or Cheez Doodles. Then next time you grab for the Cheez Doodles, ask yourself this Magic Question. Now, can you put the Cheez Doodles back?

If you happen to really love apples, find another healthy food for this question. Getting in touch with your pig-out triggers will help you to avoid overindulging in that moment of weakness.

CONCLUSION

Former acting U.S. surgeon general Dr. Kenneth Moritsugu says, "We doctors can talk until we're blue in the face about the fact that two out of three Americans are now obese or overweight. But only you as an individual have the power to decide whether or not you're going to eat fruits or cookies."

Peggy Jensen concludes by suggesting, "Put a positive spin on your food choices. Rather than grieving for doughnuts, it's all about finding tasty fruits and vegetables that you really like."

And asking yourself the right questions.

THE 10 BEST RESOURCES

Campbell, T. Colin, and Thomas M. Campbell. *The China Study: The Most Comprehensive Study of Nutrition Ever Conducted and the Startling Implications for Diet, Weight Loss and Long-term Health.* Dallas, TX: Benbella Books, 2005.

Esselstyn, Caldwell B. *Prevent and Reverse Heart Disease: The Revolutionary, Scientifically Proven, Nutrition-Based Cure.* New York: Penguin Group, 2007.

Lillien, Lisa. *Hungry Girl: Recipes and Survival Strategies for Guilt-Free Eating in the Real World.* New York: St. Martin's Press, 2008.

Mayo Clinic. "Food & Nutrition Center." www.mayoclinic.com/health/food-and-nutrition/NU99999.

MedicineNet. "Nutrition Glossary." www.medicinenet.com/script/main/art.asp?articlekey=10366.

National Heart Lung and Blood Institute. "Be Heart Smart! Eat Foods Lower in Saturated Fat and Cholesterol." http://nhlbisupport.com/chd1/Tipsheets/resourceroom.htm.

Oz, Mehmet, and Michael F. Roizen. *You: On a Diet: The Owner's Manual for Waist Management.* New York: Free Press, 2006.

Pollan, Michael. *In Defense of Food: An Eater's Manifesto.* New York: Penguin Press, 2008.

Schlosser, Eric. *Fast Food Nation.* New York: Harper Perennial, 2005.

Zinczenko, David, and Matt Goulding. *Eat This Not That! Thousands of Simple Food Swaps That Can Save You 10, 20, 30 Pounds—or More!* Emmaus, PA: Rodale, 2007.

CHAPTER 17: THE 10 BEST QUESTIONS

To Find a Great Gym or Fitness Club

> So I said to the gym instructor, "Can you teach me to do
> the splits?" He said, "How flexible are you?" I said, "I
> can't make Tuesdays."
>
> —Tim Vine, comedian

The fibromyalgia experts and longtime patients agree that becoming physically fit and exercising regularly with a combination of stretching and endurance activities is essential to managing your symptoms.

Mayo Clinic's director of Complementary and Integrative Medicine Program Dr. Brent A. Bauer advises, "Gentle, graded, consistent exercise seems to be a fundamental component of most successful management strategies. Many patients with fibromyalgia 'swing' from extreme to extreme. On really bad days, they don't do any activity. On days when they feel better, they often try to 'catch up' and then overdo it."

As fibromyalgia expert Dr. Kim Dupree Jones adds, "Exercise is an integral component of a healthy lifestyle whether or not you have fibromyalgia. You need to get more meaningful exercise into your life."

Martha Beck, well-known fibromyalgia patient, life coach, and bestselling author, agrees, "Once I got the diagnosis, I learned that what I had was real and it's not fatal. Even though it hurts a lot to exercise, exercise is actually good for it. I literally went from the doctor's to the gym. I overdid it and ended up in bed again. But I kept returning for a combination of getting to know my body and progressively asking it to become stronger and stronger."

This may seem difficult if you are in pain. But many longtime fibromyalgia patients sing the praises of exercise. Fibromyalgia sufferer and 1960s singer and songwriter Rosie Hamlin says, "Many people don't want to exercise when they are in a lot of pain. But you can just do five minutes and another ten minutes later. This will help you keep in mind that exercise will really help."

Maryland-based career coach Linda Pütz enthusiastically agrees. "I discovered that exercise is my number one pain control and sleep benefit. The absolute number one. With fibro, our bodies lie to us; it's like my body is constantly whispering, 'I'm sore and tired, the best thing to do is sit around and rest all day.' But I have to ignore that message and just get going. I always feel so much better after exercising as long as I don't overdo it. Abby MacLean, a Virginia-based information systems engineer with fibromyalgia joins the chorus. She says, "Exercise, exercise, exercise (without overdoing and hurting oneself). Water exercise is great. Keep going and don't just sit around. The worst thing you can do is to stop moving."

Belonging to a gym or fitness club (the terms are used interchangeably here) can be a great way to get and stay motivated for exercise. Yoga, tai chi, warm water therapy, strength training with light weights, and walking are recommended options for fibromyalgia patients. High impact aerobic exercise classes, stair-stepping machines, and jogging may aggravate your symptoms. Look for exercise classes for seniors if you are unsure about which program to join.

Regularly scheduled, structured exercise will also boost your self-confidence. As Harvard University assistant professor Dr. Daniel Forman says, "People who start exercising on their own in a random way are usually the ones who find less value in their exercise routines and end up stopping. Supervised people do much better."

Having a comfortable place to go that supports your fitness goals will help you keep on track. And you might even have fun.

Get guidance from your doctor before starting any exercise or joining a gym. Then if you want to explore a fitness club or gym membership, ask the membership director or another representative the following Best Questions while you are touring their fitness facility.

THE QUESTION DOCTOR SAYS:

Try to tour several local fitness centers before you make your final decision. Make extra copies of these Best Questions so that you can ask questions at each facility and compare answers later.

>>>THE 10 BEST QUESTIONS
To Find a Great Gym or Fitness Club

1. What activities and support services are available here?

This is ultimately the deal-breaker question. If you want water aerobic classes but there's no pool in this fitness club, you'll have to look elsewhere. You may want yoga classes, tai chi, massages, or walking programs but this club only offers kickboxing and step aerobics.

Follow-up questions include, "May I see a class schedule?" "What services do you offer for seniors or that are less intense?"

Also check to see if any of this club's advertised activities have additional charges or hidden fees. Some popular classes like yoga may cost extra.

2. Where is the gym located?

A key consideration in choosing a fitness club is its location. The ideal travel time is fifteen minutes or less. Make sure that parking won't send you off to the Dairy Queen in frustration.

Bill Sonnemaker, MS, an international award-winning master personal trainer and the CEO of Catalyst Fitness in Atlanta, advises, "The closer and easier it is to get to, the less likely you'll be to come up with an excuse for not going regularly. Make your drive as short as possible so you can't use the excuse, 'There's not enough time to exercise.'"

3. When is the gym open?

Check the hours to make sure they are easy to fit into your schedule. Decide for yourself what time of day you are most likely to use the facility.

Come back unannounced on another day during your preferred time to see how crowded the gym is and to check out en route traffic conditions.

4. Are the staff members degreed and certified?

Dr. Larry Hamm, a cardiac rehabilitation specialist at George Washington University, warns, "Most of the fitness clubs, not all, but most clubs hire personal trainers who are only minimally qualified without requiring any kind of college degree or a degree in exercise science or exercise physiology."

One quality check is to ask if this facility belongs to a professional fitness association, such as IDEA (www.ideafit.com) or IHRSA (www.ihrsa.org). Make sure the staff's personal certifications are from an accredited organization discussed in chapter 18.

5. How old is the equipment?

Do you see any equipment with "Out of Service" signs? Ask how often the equipment is cleaned for health and safety purposes.

6. How well designed and maintained is this facility?

The group exercise floor should be designed to provide shock absorption. Look for instructions conveniently posted for each piece of equipment. Are there enough machines so that you won't have to wait to use them? Is there enough space between machines so that you don't bump into other people? Is the pool area clean and easily accessible?

Are there gathering areas where people can sit and socialize? Is the facility bright and cheerful and the noise level tolerable?

7. How clean and comfortable is the locker room?

Check out the locker room area for cleanliness and roominess, a comfortable temperature, and good lighting. Are there any dangerous areas, such as loose tiles or carpet edges, that could cause a fall? Are towels, soap, and shampoo provided or can you obtain them for an extra charge? Is there a shower stall with wheelchair accessibility?

8. Has anyone ever been hurt here? What emergency procedures do you have in place?

You may not get an honest answer, but ask anyway. Also ask if this facility carries liability insurance in case you get injured.

The entire staff should have completed cardiopulmonary resuscitation (CPR) training at bare minimum. Ask the staff what they would do if someone had a heart attack on their premises. If they don't say, "call 911 immediately," don't go there.

9. What are the terms of the contract?

Don't get roped into an extended contract, especially if you aren't sure how committed you are at this point. There shouldn't be any pressure to sign anything, especially a long-term agreement. Ask if you can try the club for a couple of weeks or start with a month-to-month membership.

Other good follow-up questions include, "Are there any services, classes, or amenities that cost extra?" "Will the club offer a trial membership or waive the initiation fee?" "What is your cancellation policy (and any penalties)?"

Price depends on geographic location and how nice the facility is. Decide on your price range ahead of time. Most facilities charge between $30 and $50 or more per month.

Assess later if this facility seemed more service oriented or sales oriented. Bill Sonnemaker, MS, explains, "The staff should encourage you to *use* the facility, not just belong."

10. What is the atmosphere and "personality" of this fitness club?

Paige Waehner, a certified personal trainer and author in Chicago, says, "You want to feel comfortable in your workout environment. If you walk in and the music is too loud, the floor is very crowded, or you feel overwhelmed by all the machines and gadgets, you'll be less likely to show up for your workouts."

Look around and decide if the clients are people who you can relate to. Do they look happy or stressed out? Socializing at a fitness club will keep you coming back because you develop workout buddy friendships.

How many people are working with personal trainers? Do the trainers look bored or are they actively engaged? Bill Sonnemaker,

MS, says, "The bottom line here is when you walk into a club you should feel comfortable as if you belong there."

❯ The Magic Question

Does this facility belong to the Medical Fitness Association?

Perhaps you've never heard of medical fitness centers because there's not one on every street corner. Dr. Cary Wing, executive director of the Medical Fitness Association, explains, "By definition, a medical fitness center must have either a medical director or a physician advisory board that oversees the program, although the supervision may not be full time."

Most medical fitness centers are affiliated with a hospital, health care system, or physicians' practices. They differ from regular gyms because the staff is made up of exercise physiologists, physical therapists, or athletic trainers with nationally recognized certification and experience in helping people who are medically challenged.

This is good news and an extra measure of safety for you. These facilities are more likely to do an initial full health risk assessment, taking your fibromyalgia history and other medical conditions into consideration; require higher standards of qualifications and performance from their staff; and understand your exercise limitations.

There are currently about 950 medical fitness centers in the United States, with the numbers growing to meet the health needs of an aging population. See their Web site at www.medicalfitness .org.

CONCLUSION

You can incorporate pain-busting exercise into your life, save money, and ensure your health and safety are in good hands by asking the right questions before joining a fitness club or gym. Get your doctor's approval first. Then look for a facility that matches your needs and style. As Dr. Cary Wing says, "There's an intimidation factor in a fitness center for many people."

No matter how fancy a health club is, your ultimate Best Question is, "Will I keep coming back?" Paige Waehner concludes, "Ask yourself if this is a place you can see yourself going to on a regular basis." All the latest equipment, the nicest showers, or the world's best personal trainers won't do you a bit of good if you don't actually use the facility.

THE 10 BEST RESOURCES

American Council on Exercise. "Exercise and Fibromyalgia." www
.acefitness.org/fitfacts/pdfs/fitfacts/itemid_89.pdf.

American Council on Exercise. "How to Choose a Health Club." www
.acefitness.org/fitfacts/fitfacts_display.aspx?itemid=111.

American Council on Exercise. "Work Out Chronic Fatigue." www
.acefitness.org/fitfacts/fitfacts_display.aspx?itemid=26.

American Pain Foundation. "Chair Yoga for Good Living." www
.painfoundation.org/ManageYourPain/Yoga/yogabooklet.pdf.

American Physical Therapy Association. "Find a PT." www.apta.org/AM/
Template.cfm?Section=Find_a_PT3&Template=/APTAAPPS/FindAPT/
findaptsearch.cfm.

Crotzer, Shoosh Lettick. *Yoga for Fibromyalgia: Move, Breathe, and Relax to Improve Your Quality of Life.* Berkeley, CA: Rodmell Press, 2008.

Fibromyalgia Information Foundation. "Exercise Advice." www.myalgia .com/Exercise%20advice.htm.

Fibromyalgia Information Foundation. "FM-specific Exercise DVDs." www.myalgia.com.

National Fibromyalgia Association. "Exercise." www.fmaware.org/site/ PageServer?pagename=topics_exercise.

Rosenstein, Ann A. *Water Exercises for Fibromyalgia: The Gentle Way to Relax and Reduce Pain.* Enumclaw, WA: Idyll Arbor, 2006.

CHAPTER 18: THE 10 BEST QUESTIONS
To Hire a Top Personal Trainer

I really don't think I need buns of steel. I'd be happy with buns of cinnamon.

—Ellen DeGeneres

Having a personal trainer who understands your exercise needs and physical limitations can be a wonderful motivation to keep moving. A study published in the *British Medical Journal* concluded that people with fibromyalgia who worked with a personal trainer twice a week for twelve weeks were twice as likely to report feeling "much better" than those people who didn't participate.

However, award-winning personal trainer Bill Sonnemaker, MS, warns, "Over 95 percent of people practicing as personal trainers should not be doing so because they are not certified by an accredited and medically recognized organization." Like any other profession, personal fitness training attracts its share of losers. In fact, trainers' missing credentials are often ignored, especially if they look like bodybuilding rock stars.

Ask the following Best Questions when you interview potential personal trainers and before you sign a contract. Make sure you get someone who will help—not hurt—you.

>>> THE 10 BEST QUESTIONS
To Hire a Top Personal Trainer

1. Are you certified by an accredited organization? If so, which one?

There are over three hundred personal trainer certification programs, but only four are fully accredited. These are the National Academy of Sports Medicine (NASM), the American Council on Exercise (ACE), the National Strength and Conditioning Association (NACA), and the American College of Sports Medicine (ACSM). Don't be fooled by the others.

2. How long have you been a personal trainer?

You want someone who has enough experience to anticipate your needs and safety issues, yet isn't so burned out that they only chitchat while you sweat it out on a treadmill. Experience is no guarantee, but it helps.

3. What experience and education do you have for working with people with fibromyalgia or chronic pain?

Ask about her specific training (course names and dates) and the specific information (how long together, how many sessions, and how long ago) for her clients like you. Check her general understanding of fibromyalgia or ask about prior experience working with mobility-challenged elderly people.

4. When is the last time you completed a continuing education course? Did you take this class online or with a live instructor?

The best fitness instructors complete a minimum of twenty training hours every two years and take live classes rather than online correspondence courses. Ideally, your trainer also has some college education, preferably a bachelor's degree in exercise physiology.

5. How do you plan to personalize my training program?

Avoid someone who has a cookie-cutter approach to exercise. A personal trainer should emphasize establishing a doable and fun routine. Two red flags are a lack of interest in you personally and a lack of questions about your goals.

6. How will you help me to meet my fitness goals?

Make sure your training plan is gentle enough to accommodate flare-ups yet challenging enough to break a little sweat on your better days. Another quality indicator is a personal trainer who is well organized and will keep notes on your progress.

7. What is your follow-up strategy?

The best personal trainers anticipate the day you'll leave them to exercise independently on your own. To accomplish this, they typically give "homework" exercises on printed handouts for you to do in-between your workout sessions together.

8. Do you have professional liability insurance?

This matters because it shows a higher level of professionalism and protects you in case you get hurt and it's the trainer's fault.

9. What are your hourly rates? Do you have any discounts or other offers? Can I try a sample session for free?

Rates vary according to geographic location and a trainer's qualifications, ranging between $50 and $100 or more per hour. Keep in mind that the cheapest trainer in town may not be able to help you reach your goals. Some offer a free trial session.

10. Could you please give me the names and contact details for three of your clients that I can check with?

Ask for referrals to other people with pain issues and not teenage track stars or professional athletes. Then really follow through on your calls.

When you call ask: "Why did you like this trainer?" "Was there ever a time that you questioned his judgment about your safety or well-being?" and "Would you send your friends or family to this trainer?" These referrals can be a wealth of information.

❯ The Magic Question

How do you plan to stay in communication with my doctor? How often?

Bill Sonnemaker, MS, says, "It's important that the trainer has immediate interaction with the physician. A really savvy trainer will have either an e-mail or fax communications going on with the doctor that includes telling the doctor [or physical therapist] about the training program and what types of exercises we are proposing."

Chicago-based certified trainer Paige Waehner adds, "You want to make sure your trainer is willing to reach out and accept help and guidance from other resources including your doctor or physical therapist."

THE QUESTION DOCTOR SAYS:

In addition to reflecting on how this trainer reacted to your questions, also consider how many questions he asked you. Did he ask these questions with genuine interest and listen intently or did he just seem to be going through the motions? Does this person understand pain? This little insight might say a lot about how likely this trainer is to go the extra mile for you.

CONCLUSION

If you are trying to incorporate more physical activity in your life, a personal trainer can keep you motivated and organized in meeting your exercise goals. However, you don't want a muscle-bound beach bum who's just masquerading as a personal trainer.

Working with a credentialed, experienced trainer can help you to internalize a lifelong commitment to getting more physical activity despite the challenges of living with fibromyalgia.

Verify your exercise goals with your doctor before you start with any independent program or trainer. And keep checking to make sure your personal trainer and doctor are still communicating regularly about your progress.

THE 10 BEST RESOURCES

American College of Sports Medicine. "Selecting and Effectively Using a Personal Trainer." www.acsm.org/AM/Template.cfm?Section=Brochures 2&Template=/CM/ContentDisplay.cfm&ContentID=8103.

American Council on Exercise. "Fit Facts: Choosing Fitness Trainers and Instructors." www.acefitness.org/fitfacts/default.aspx#Choosing%20 Fitness%20Trainers%20and%20Instructors.

American Council on Exercise. "How to Choose an Online Personal Trainer." www.acefitness.org/fitfacts/fitfacts_display.aspx?itemid=116.

American Council on Exercise. "How to Choose the Right Personal Trainer." www.acefitness.org/fitfacts/fitfacts_display.aspx?itemid=19.

Aquatic Exercise Association. "H20 Personal Training." www.aeawave .com/PublicPages/Home/tabid/54/ctl/DetailView/mid457/itemid/110/ Default.aspx.

Catalyst Fitness. "Choosing a Personal Trainer." www.fitnesscatalyst.com/ Choosing-a-Personal-Trainer.html.

International Council on Active Aging. "How to Select an Age-Friendly Personal Fitness Trainer." www.icaa.cc/facilitylocator/icaapftguide.pdf.

National Strength and Conditioning Association. "Find a Trainer." www .nsca-lift.org.

Waehner, Paige. About.com. "Choosing a Personal Trainer." http:// exercise.about.com/cs/forprofessionals/a/choosetrainer.htm.

Waehner, Paige. About.com. "Why a Trainer May be Right for You." http://exercise.about.com/cs/forprofessionals/a/choosetrainer.htm.

PART IV:

Building Your Future Life and Good Relationships

The last section of this book addresses your emotional, loving, sexual, intimate, social, and spiritual needs as you battle fibromyalgia. Each chapter offers the Best Questions to ask yourself or others in your search for a happier future despite your illness.

Many people dealing with chronic pain and fatigue experience a rocky rollercoaster ride of emotions and depression. If this sounds familiar, see chapter 19.

Relationships are often strained when someone has a chronic illness, especially an "invisible" disease like fibromyalgia. There's often guilt, blame, and misunderstandings between partners. In chapter 20 find the actual script to help you and your partner talk more easily. In essence, these Best Questions give you "permission" to have this often difficult conversation.

Likewise, use chapter 21 to talk with your partner about your sexual and intimate needs, another often taboo topic. Chapter 22 is a dress rehearsal for talking with your children about your fibromyalgia, while chapter 23 helps you decide who you want to tell about your illness. See chapter 24 to make a well-informed decision about joining a support group, either as a person with fibromyalgia or for help with other medical conditions.

Most people with fibromyalgia can benefit from exploring their financial health, as discussed in chapter 25. The 10 Worst Questions in chapter 26 are partly just for fun and also to illustrate that even well-intended friends and family members may not know what to say to you. The book concludes with chapter 27's Best Questions to get in deeper touch with your spiritual health, which is often in crisis due to the burden of living with a chronic illness.

The Question Doctor sincerely hopes these Best Questions will serve you well as your companion and guide as you redefine your future, renew your relationships, and find inner peace about your health challenges.

CHAPTER 19

THE 10 BEST QUESTIONS

For Your Emotional Health After

Fibromyalgia

Feelings are much like waves. We can't stop them from
coming but we can choose which one to surf.

—Jonatan Mårtensson

Having fibromyalgia often feels like a ride on an emotional roller coaster. It's difficult not to feel frustrated, disappointed, stressed out, depressed, and angry about life when you are tired or in pain all the time.

Lynne Matallana, the president of the National Fibromyalgia Association advises, "The emotional side of things is very important." Dr. Daniel J. Clauw, a fibromyalgia expert at the University of Michigan, agrees, "It is very common for patients with fibromyalgia to develop depression, anxiety, and other emotional problems."

On top of feeling physically lousy, you may have to cope with many people (including some doctors) who don't understand or don't believe that you are really sick. Your income, relationships with loved ones, and quality of life have probably been profoundly affected by your loss of independence. You may have experienced actual grief over these losses without exactly realizing it. Prolonged negative emotions and chronic stress can trigger worsening fibromyalgia symptoms, especially sleeplessness and fatigue.

Ask yourself the following Best Questions to clarify your feelings, tap into this important mind-body connection, and hopefully find peace of mind. There's no judgment here and no right or wrong answers, only degrees of emotional honesty or dishonesty with yourself. Share your answers with others only if you want to.

>>>THE 10 BEST QUESTIONS
For Your Emotional Health After Fibromyalgia

1. What was my emotional state before my fibromyalgia symptoms started?

One way to recover your sense of balance is to reflect on who you were and define your emotional state before chronic pain and fatigue became routine. Maybe you were overstressed in a dead-end job, arguing constantly with your defiant teenager, or barely hanging on to a rocky marriage. Or life was good, full of raising children, church activities, and travel adventures.

Think of this question as an emotional audit and a reality check. Be honest with yourself to avoid mourning the "good old days"—which may not have been quite as great as you remember.

2. What coping strategies have been most successful for me in the past?

Before now, what were your greatest emotional and personal challenges? How did you handle them? What did you do especially well and feel most proud about?

Analyze your past successes so that you can start from a position of personal strength. Get out your past coping strategies, take a look at them, shine them up, accentuate the positive, and use them again.

3. How do I feel about my body's changes?

Living with constant pain can make you more reflective about how your body has changed (or betrayed) you. Some people with fibromyalgia start a journal (or a blog) of everything that is happening to them—what the doctors say, about treatments, and tips they learned from Web sites or books. Others prefer to keep a personal log about their feelings, relationships, spiritual thoughts or prayers, hopes, dreams, and reasons for gratitude.

If you like this idea, find your own way of journaling (or start a blog). Try to write something every day without self-criticism, editing, or treating it as another chore. You can tell your story with pictures and photographs, too. For more ideas, go to Caring-Bridge (www.caringbridge.org).

4. How well am I handling other people's reactions to my fibromyalgia?

How other people, especially loved ones, treat you and your "invisible" disease probably affects you a lot, especially if you must often "defend" or explain your illness to others. Family members and friends can be very supportive or crush you with finger-pointing judgments that cause additional emotional hardships.

For example, if a brother freaks out about your illness, it's only human nature to absorb and react with fear, too. Maybe your self-centered sister angers you because all she cares about is not having fibromyalgia herself.

Perhaps your partner treats you like a breakable glass doll or is often withdrawn and sullen. His or her reaction can anger you or make you feel helpless.

Others may pull away from you, blame you for causing your "mysterious" disease, or act like nothing is wrong. Unexpected reactions from others can cause you to become depressed, stressed out, or angry, especially if you don't have an outlet to discuss your feelings. See chapter 23.

5. Where can I get help? Who are my best resources for support?

Talk to your family doctor, specialist, support group, family, friends, or a trusted religious leader about getting help. Don't be afraid to ask for help or actively seek it out. As fibromyalgia expert Dr. Michael McNett says, "Fibromyalgia patients need a lot of emotional support."

You deserve support and comfort as you deal with this chronic illness. Many people, and especially women, are better at giving care to others than asking for and receiving help for themselves. But if you don't take care of yourself, you may jeopardize your future health and well-being.

THE QUESTION DOCTOR SAYS:

In psychiatrist Dr. Elisabeth Kübler-Ross's 1969 groundbreaking book *On Death and Dying,* she outlined five stages of grief as the pattern most people experience as they face a chronic illness or deal with grief:
1. **Shock and denial.** "This can't be happening to me."
2. **Anger.** "Why me? This isn't fair. I want my own life, too."
3. **Bargaining.** "Just let me live through another day."
4. **Depression.** "Why even bother anymore?"
5. **Acceptance.** "I'm going to be okay and live through this."
   Not everyone moves neatly through the stages in an orderly fashion or at the same pace. For example, you might experience anger (stage 2) and then depression (stage 4), go backward to denial (stage 1), or get stuck at bargaining (stage 3).
   The next five Best Questions use Dr. Kübler-Ross's stages to help you get in touch with your emotional responses to your fibromyalgia.

6. What am I denying or avoiding about my fibromyalgia? (Stage 1)

Many people cope with chronic pain and insomnia by pretending it isn't happening. But this coping strategy may be costing you lots of your limited energy that could be better used for proactive approaches to alternative treatments, like taking a water aerobics or yoga class.

What matters the most is how well you cope emotionally with your illness and that you take proactive steps toward positive lifestyle changes, including more exercise and a better diet. You must conquer denial before you can be a fully successful patient.

7. How can I channel my anger into a positive healing experience? (Stage 2)

Nearly everyone goes through this stage. Most people with fibromyalgia feel like their lives have been hijacked by their disease. How could my body betray me like this?

Gregg Piburn, a Colorado management consultant and author of the book, *Beyond Chaos: One Man's Journey Alongside His Chronically Ill Wife,* says, "Everyone is angry at the situation but sometimes that spills over into anger at each other." You may be angry at yourself, other family members, your doctors, or God.

Fibromyalgia shouldn't happen to nice people. Try to channel your anger into positive actions, like researching this disease and slowing down your hectic life to smell the roses.

It's very important to move beyond this stage. The people who get stuck here increase their odds for having a heart attack. Dr. Hamilton Beazley, author of the book *No Regrets,* says, "You have to look for the lessons and the gifts. But you can't do that until you get over the anger. Every tragedy brings lessons."

Get professional help if your anger is out of control. Whatever you do, don't stay angry forever.

8. What am I bargaining for either consciously or unconsciously? (Stage 3)

Dr. Kübler-Ross describes this stage in her book, *On Death and Dying*:

> Bargaining is really an attempt to postpone; it has to include a prize offered "for good behavior," it also sets a self-imposed deadline . . . like children who say, "I will never fight with my sister again."

Does this sound familiar? Maybe you've had fleeting thoughts of all the good things you'll do for yourself and family if God just lets you get through the pain. Fear is a major component of bargaining and plays a key (and unconscious) role in your choice of treatments.

Bargaining is another dangerous place to get stuck. It can lead to an endless loop of failing to meet your own self-imposed high standards or expectations that cause subsequent despair.

9. How can I better cope with my feelings of being stressed out and depressed? (Stage 4)

Dr. Richard Stoltz, the director for military and family health at the National Naval Medical Center in Bethesda, Maryland, comments, "The failure to acknowledge the potential difficulties of adjusting to changes can contribute to a person becoming overwhelmed."

Seattle-based fibromyalgia expert, Dr. Patrick Wood, offers more wisdom, "I think there's a risk in thinking that fibromyalgia is just an abnormal type of depression. Anxiety is a much more common part of living with fibromyalgia than 'depressiveness.' Anxiousness has a great impact on the daily functioning of fibromyalgia patients. It's not unusual for anyone with a chronic, disabling condition to become discouraged."

You can move beyond depression by proactively arming yourself with medical knowledge about fibromyalgia and making healthy lifestyle changes. Seek professional help if you have suicidal thoughts, your depression persists more than two weeks, or you have no one to talk with. See more on stress in chapter 15.

10. What steps can I take to accept my fibromyalgia? (Stage 5)

Dr. Kübler-Ross believed that it's the acknowledgment of loss that holds the key to acceptance with dignity and grace. Another version of this Best Question is, "How can I treat myself with more compassion?"

Acceptance and self-love can help you overcome your internal critic who only remembers your former ability to win dance contests, have great sex, or play basketball. Guilt drains your energy to make positive adjustments.

❯ The Magic Question

How can I feel my best today?

Many persons with fibromyalgia allow their illness, external circumstances, or other people to determine how they feel. You can take back control of your feelings with this Magic Question. It puts you in the driver's seat rather than being a passive victim of fibromyalgia.

Your renewed sense of self-worth and confidence for living are priceless. Start each day with this Magic Question to find your own emotional well-being, self-acceptance, and a sense of inner peace.

CONCLUSION

A diagnosis of fibromyalgia can be emotionally transformative and a powerful wake-up call to examine your feelings, coping skills, relationships, and yourself.

Having this chronic illness can flood you with complex and changing emotions that are rarely acknowledged or discussed. But they matter. Patty Wooten of Santa Cruz, California, is a cardiac nurse who specializes in the therapeutic benefits of humor. She says, "Emotions can have a toxic effect on the body, like anger, hostility, stress, hopelessness, and depression. When we live with these emotions all the time, they create chemical changes in the body that actually weaken the immune system."

Don't hesitate to ask for help. There are many resources available from your doctors, the Internet, in this book, or in other books. The bottom line is: **You are not alone.**

THE 10 BEST RESOURCES

Amen, Daniel G. *Change Your Brain, Change Your Life: The Breakthrough Program for Conquering Anxiety, Depression, Obsessiveness, Anger, and Impulsiveness.* New York: Three Rivers Press, 1999.

Boss, Pauline. *Ambiguous Loss: Learning to Live with Unresolved Grief.* Cambridge: Harvard University Press, 2000.

Kübler-Ross, Elisabeth. *On Grief and Grieving: Finding the Meaning of Grief Through the Five Stages of Loss.* New York: Simon & Schuster, 2005.

Lewis & Clark College. "Grieving the Losses Caused by Fibromyalgia." http://www.lclark.edu/~sherrons/topic_context.htm.

Mayo Clinic. "Denial: Overcome Denial by Taking Action and Moving Forward." www.mayoclinic.com/health/denial/SR00043.

Moyers, Bill. *Healing and the Mind*. New York: Main Street Books, 1995.

National Fibromyalgia Association. "Depression and Fibromyalgia." http://www.fmaware.org/site/News2?page=NewsArticle&id=6229.

National Fibromyalgia Association. "Fibromyalgia: After the Diagnosis . . ." http://www.fmaware.org/site/News2?page=NewsArticle& id=6313.

WebMD. "Fibromyalgia Tips for Coping." http://www.webmd.com/ fibromyalgia/guide/fibromyalgia-tips-for-coping.

Williams, J. Mark G., John D. Teasdale, Zindel V. Segal, and Jon Kabat-Zinn. *The Mindful Way Through Depression: Freeing Yourself from Chronic Unhappiness*. New York: Guilford Press, 2007.

CHAPTER 20: THE 10 BEST QUESTIONS

When Talking with Your Partner
About Fibromyalgia

Marriages are all happy. It's having breakfast together that
causes all the trouble.

—Irish proverb

Fibromyalgia profoundly affects relationships, marriages,
and long-term partnerships. Being in constant pain and disabled can magnify a relationship's past imperfections or
strengthen what was already strong between partners.

Fibromyalgia expert, Dr. Michael McNett, explains, "Fibromyalgia polarizes relationships. One partner's fibromyalgia can
expand fissures that had been almost invisible; but sometimes the
diagnosis can bring couples closer together."

Gregg Piburn, a Colorado management consultant and the author of *Beyond Chaos: One Man's Journey Alongside His Chronically Ill
Wife,* says, "Struggling with chronic illness in the family was very
difficult for us. I call fibromyalgia the 'Intruder' because it robs
your relationship. I think we got better as time went on, but our
kids watched us struggle and we made mistakes."

Shifting roles in the partnership can cause communication
breakdowns. The well spouse is suddenly thrust into the role of
caregiver or must take on additional chores. A key difference between men and women is their comfort level with the role of caregiver. Some men find caregiving unfamiliar and awkward territory
because they are accustomed to solving problems. Men typically
prefer to be Mr. Fix-it. Some male partners get frustrated with the

permanence of fibromyalgia's symptoms. Unfortunately, the divorce rate among couples touched by chronic illness is a whopping 75 percent according to a national survey cited by Rest Ministries (www.restministries.org).

Daily routines can be heaved upside down. Both partners often feel tremendous stress, usually within their relationship as well as from external stressors, such as countless doctor appointments, new medications, overbooked schedules, and financial worries.

The goal of this chapter is to help you and your partner communicate more effectively by asking each other Best Questions. These questions will work in either direction—the person with fibromyalgia asking the partner and vice versa. These questions also work well for couples in lesbian or gay relationships. Revisit these Best Questions over time to understand your evolving needs or how your relationship is changing.

THE QUESTION DOCTOR SAYS

How you ask your questions is just as important in a close relationship as *what* you ask each other. Let this chapter give you "permission" to ask each other the tough questions that you might have avoided or may not have known to ask otherwise.

Your attitude and timing are critical to a successful conversation. Plan a time to talk when you are both relaxed. Use the questions in whatever order works best for you or add your own. Take a time-out when needed or if you become upset while talking.

›››THE 10 BEST QUESTIONS
When Talking with Your Partner About Fibromyalgia

1. When were we most successful in communicating with each other in the past? How can we use the same methods now to deal with this illness together?

Fibromyalgia is like an uninvited houseguest that's here to stay. Your current communications may be hampered by unspoken feelings of anxiety, anger, or anguish about the daily reality of living with fibromyalgia.

A positive start is to reflect on the past good times. Talk over these times and remember how well you communicated.

Longtime partners often assume they can read each other's minds. This can be a fatal flaw and shut down good listening. Talk in specifics with frequent "I" and "we" statements ("I think we should . . . ," "I feel we need to consider . . ."). Use openers like, "I hear you saying . . . ," "Is that right?" or "Tell me more." Keep your facial expressions open and your body language positive.

Harriette Cole, author of the nationally syndicated advice column, *Sense and Sensitivity,* and a creative director for *Ebony* magazine, suggests: "It's best in the beginning to ask welcoming questions. Do your best not to be hostile, condescending, or doubting. . . . Ask your questions honestly and without judgment and not like an inquisition."

A MESSAGE FROM MARS AND VENUS

Dr. John Gray, relationship guru and author of the best-selling *Men Are from Mars, Women Are from Venus* book series, says, "The biggest problem between men and women is this. She gives an answer and he assumes there's a period and that's the end of the point. That's never the end of the point; she's just warming up."

2. What areas of our lives must we maintain to ensure as much normalcy as possible?

You need a cocoon of normalcy in order to function on a daily basis. Author and psychotherapist Rachael Freed says, "Everyone outside the patient wants 'normal' to return because it's so threatening for them."

But having a chronic illness becomes the "new normal." As fibromyalgia expert at Oregon Health and Science University, Dr. Kim Dupree Jones, states, "Most people who get fibromyalgia start to get it in their thirties or forties during their most productive years in the workplace and raising families."

Well spouse Gregg Piburn advises, "For the partner, chronic illness can become like an ongoing spectatorship. It's no longer *our* problem; it's *her* problem. It's very important to band together and see the 'Intruder' as a common enemy. If both partners open up while in the foxhole of the war against the 'Intruder,' they can't help but become tighter as a couple."

Solve your problems together. Your life and household responsibilities must continue, but decide which ones are critical needs (like paying the bills) and which ones are the "wants" (continuing your daughter's flute lessons). The daily bottom-line question, "What's for dinner?" isn't going away.

Normalcy also soothes frazzled nerves and the raw edges of relationships. For example, keep up e-mail correspondence with long-distance friends or an online support group.

3. What role changes in our partnership do we need to make to get through this thing together?

Your past roles and the division of labor in your partnership may now be turned upside down. In essence, you have two new job descriptions to write. This is a critical task that should not be overlooked.

Couples' misunderstandings or unspoken assumptions about roles are a breeding ground for festering guilt, resentments, and even lifelong animosities toward each other. Clarify your expectations for each other. The well partner may need to cook or do more household chores. Longtime fibromyalgia patient Dot Gerecke in Horsham, Australia, advises, "Ask for help with the chores, especially on your 'off days.'"

4. What has this been like for you?

This simple question may uncover a hornet's nest of complaints, a flood of feelings, or no new information at all. It's only understandable that some people who live with constant pain can overlook their partners' feelings and experiences.

Dr. Kim Dupree Jones, explains, "It's so hard for the spouse because the person with fibromyalgia can no longer do many of the things that they once enjoyed together, like sports, running, and other physical activities." Gregg Piburn agrees with his story, "In the 1970s, I bought Sherrie running shoes and cross-country skis. In the 1980s, I bought her a recliner chair and cordless phone."

Relationship advisers Dr. Scott Peck and Shannon Peck of Solana Beach, California, comment, "There are many ways to bring the empowering combination of kindness and love into your marriage. One way is to ask simple, direct questions."

This Best Question works well for many occasions, so ask it often.

5. How can we help each other deal with the stress in our lives?

You may be facing a double-dose stress whammy. Chronic illness strains even the best relationships.

Many couples experience internal misunderstandings, self-pity, anger, and financial and sexual problems. The ill partner may become disabled. All of this is added to the pressure cooker of routine work, family, and financial demands.

Maryland licensed clinical social worker Mark Gorkin says, "Caregivers frequently cycle between anger, due to the unreasonable demands of caregiving, and being in a state of chronic guilt and stress for not being able to do it all."

The only way out is to work together as a team. Identify what's causing each of you the greatest stress and then talk over what you can practically do to alleviate some of it. Some friends or family members might gladly help out, too.

6. How can I show you that I love you?

Welcome to the "Hugs Department." There's an old saying that "hugs are the universal medicine." Even if you are struggling in this relationship, saying, "I love you," or giving small tokens of your affection can mean the world to either partner.

7. How can we still enjoy being together and have fun?

Don't let fibromyalgia rob you of a sense of humor and fun. Sure, you probably can't do all the things you could before, but that doesn't mean you can't do anything that's fun or at least talk about what you will do another time.

What's something silly or easy that you two can do together once in a while just like the old days? Get your favorite take-out food, watch a stupid movie together, take a walk together, or see old friends.

Being sick is no fun, but laughter can go a long way in strengthening the good glue of your relationship. See chapter 26.

8. What can I do to help you now and later?

It might just be little things, like doing household chores or errands, or helping with child care duties. Sometimes a partner secretly needs more reassurances despite putting on a brave front.

The basic gender disconnect is that women don't have much practice in asking for help and men only know how to solve problems. By asking each other this question, you can explore your true needs.

9. Do we need professional counseling or other help for our marriage?

It's a sign of strength to know when you need outside help to overcome your differences or communication breakdowns. There is nothing to be ashamed of if you decide you need marriage counseling, want to join a support group, or decide to meet with a therapist. When one partner is sick, it puts a tremendous burden on the relationship, even if it is a top-notch one.

10. What old rules do we need to break? What new rules do we need to establish?

Most relationships have unwritten but inviolable rules that govern everything from who takes the garbage out to how nutritious dinner has to be. This is the opposite of Best Question 2. Now we're talking about what you *do* want to change.

Typically, the old rules involved household chores (who does what and when), favorite routines that need acceptance or permission (Friday night poker games or shopping sprees), and the little picky stuff (neatly folded laundry).

Figure out together which rules to keep or toss to match your current circumstances. A household's unwritten and unspoken rules can be a source of unspoken assumptions, misunderstandings, and even great stress between partners. Call a truce on judging each other's past actions, wipe the slate clean, and start over as a team effort.

❯ The Magic Question

What are you afraid to ask me? What are we not talking about that needs to be addressed?

This is the all-important elephant-in-the room question where everyone present is ignoring an obvious truth and not talking about something right under their nose.

So, what is YOUR elephant? Most likely, your elephant is something you're intensely afraid of, like facing disability, lost sexual intimacy, or unspoken fears about family finances.

Unacknowledged elephants have a way of just getting bigger and bigger unless you point them out and admit to their existence. This might be a hard question to ask each other. But with the right spirit of shared hopes and dreams, it can be the most liberating question you ever ask.

CONCLUSION

Many couples enjoy being together despite living with the "Intruder." The secret is a willingness to do whatever it takes to make the relationship work and to keep the communication lines open. In fact, some couples draw closer and join forces as allies against their common enemy.

Asking each other these Best Questions and any of your own questions will clear the air. Fears, stress, and anger are best extinguished by honest sharing and "best listening" to each other.

THE 10 BEST RESOURCES

American Counseling Association. "Counselor Directory." www
.counseling.org/Resources/CounselorDirectory/TP/Home/CT2.aspx.

Chapman, Gary. *The Five Love Languages: How to Express Heartfelt
Commitment to Your Mate.* Chicago: Northfield Publishing, 1995.

Family Caregiver Alliance. "Fact Sheets & Publications." www.caregiver
.org/caregiver/jsp/publications.jsp?nodeid=345.

Gottman, John M. *The Relationship Cure: A 5 Step Guide to Strengthening
Your Marriage, Family, and Friendships.* New York: Three Rivers Press,
2002.

Gottman, John M., and Nan Silver. *The Seven Principles for Making Marriage
Work: A Practical Guide from the Country's Foremost Relationship Expert.* New
York: John Wiley & Sons, Inc., 2000.

Gray, John. *Men Are from Mars, Women Are from Venus: The Classic Guide to
Understanding the Opposite Sex.* New York: Harper Paperbacks, 2004.

Hendrix, Harville. *Getting the Love You Want: A Guide for Couples,* rev. ed.
New York: Holt Paperbacks, 2007.

National Fibromyalgia Association. "To Love, In Sickness and in Health."
www.fmaware.org/site/News2?page=NewsArticle&id=5351.

National Fibromyalgia Association. "When a Loved One Has FM—How
Can I Help?" www.fmaware.org/site/News2?page=NewsArticle&id=5350.

Piburn, Gregg. *Beyond Chaos: One Man's Journey Alongside His Chronically
Ill Wife.* Atlanta: Arthritis Foundation, 1999.

CHAPTER 21: THE 10 BEST QUESTIONS

About Sex, Intimacy, and Fibromyalgia

Whoever called it necking was a poor judge of anatomy.

—Groucho Marx

It's tough to feel sexy and be in intense pain at the same time. When one partner in an intimate relationship has fibromyalgia it creates unique challenges to overcome. Muscle aches can be aggravated during certain positions or by touching or squeezing.

Many people with fibromyalgia also battle other health problems that sap their energy, stamina, and interest in having sex. Your symptoms may cause depression and a lowered self-image, which in turn fuels more anxiety about initiating a romp in the bedroom.

However, it's still possible to explore new avenues for an intimate and sexually satisfying relationship. Medical experts suggest it helps if you accept your fibromyalgia symptoms, conquer negative emotions, such as disappointment, and use lots of pillows and patience.

The other key element to intimacy and good sex is open communication with your partner. Talk over how you can share your needs, about what works and what doesn't, and plan together for more comfortable sex.

As Dr. Julia Heiman, the executive director of the famous Kinsey Institute for Research in Sex, Gender, and Reproduction, says, "The value of asking questions for couples in intimate relationships is that it's a way of trying to see the other person as they are . . . No matter how long they've been together, that's really crucial."

Asking each other the following Best Questions can help you

to build strong communication channels for your intimate relations. These questions work equally well for either partner to ask and in gay or lesbian relationships.

THE QUESTION DOCTOR SAYS:

Some sex experts say that the most potent — and most underutilized — sex tool is your voice. Asking each other these Best Questions along with your own questions can be fun, sexy, and rebuild your confidence to be together.

Talk also with your doctor and ask for suggestions or resources. If you feel too embarrassed or shy, show him this chapter to help start the conversation. Think of these Best Questions as "permission" to be more open about tough issues.

〉〉〉THE 10 BEST QUESTIONS
About Sex, Intimacy, and Fibromyalgia

1. How can we best communicate with each other about our needs for sex and intimacy?

Women tend to romanticize about sex while men have a body-centered or recreational approach. These natural differences between men and women explain why talking about sex can be tricky.

Your best communication might be using no words at all. Simple nonverbal cues, such as a "come hither" glance or wink, help to smooth misunderstandings and clarify your amorous intentions.

2. Are you comfortable being intimate?

If you are having trouble with your sexual relations or have stopped touching, this question will help you to find out why. You can interrupt this question both literally (pain during relations) and figuratively (feeling a sense of closeness).

3. How can we redefine our intimacy and sexual pleasure needs?

If the answer to question 2 was yes, do something about it. To get in the mood, try the following:

- Enjoy a romantic candlelight dinner or get-away trip.
- Take a warm, soothing bath together.
- Offer a very gentle massage.
- Watch an erotic video together.

4. What physical changes in your body do you want me to know about?

A woman with fibromyalgia may be reluctant to talk about her pain with her partner for fear of seeming sexually diminished or unattractive. A man with fibromyalgia may fear a performance failure. Older bodies may mean less natural lubrication for women or less stamina for men. This is a gentle way to approach a tough topic.

5. What can I do to please you?

If you focus on mutual pleasure, sex becomes fun again. Intimacy is proven good medicine—for both of you.

Harriette Cole, author of the nationally syndicated advice column, *Sense and Sensitivity,* and the creative director of *Ebony* magazine, says, "I think questions are very important in all relationships, especially in intimate relationships."

6. What's the craziest or funniest thing we could do to show our love for each other?

Rediscover your passion by having fun together. Put aside your worries and fears so that you can live in this moment of passion together—again.

7. Is there anything off limits now that was okay before?

If you don't ask each other this question, your unspoken assumptions about what's acceptable and what's not can cause misunderstandings. Talk this question out without criticism, judgment, or harboring old sexual or marital problems. Be honest about what hurts.

8. We agree we both have a low interest in sex right now. What can we do to get back on track?

This Best Question applies to the times that neither of you wants sexual relations. Assuming you want to try again, this question clears the air while keeping the door open for later.

9. We can't agree about having sexual relations or being intimate. How can we work it out?

Even if you've lost sexual desire, you can still be intimate and show affection through kissing, touching, stroking, cuddling, and hugging each other, or by sharing loving words of comfort and hope.

10. Do we need professional help?

Consider the option of talking with a professional therapist or marriage counselor. Unresolved sexual tensions can result in emotional distance in long-term relationships.

❯ The Magic Question

What sexual fears are we not talking about that need to be addressed?

Not talking about sexual problems puts a tremendous strain on your relationship, just at the very time when you need closeness, good communication, and each other more than ever.

For example, fibromyalgia spouse Gregg Piburn recalls in his book, *Beyond Chaos,* "Chronic illness rocked our boat in many ways, including sexually . . . But we rarely talked about the new challenges in our sex lives."

CONCLUSION

Sex may be the last thing on your mind when you are living with chronic pain. But being intimate can make you feel loved and supported. There's also strong scientific evidence indicating that pleasurable sex and intimacy function as powerful relaxants and pain suppressants.

You don't have to give up on your joy. Find the courage to talk about it through these and your own Best Questions.

THE 10 BEST RESOURCES

ABC News. "Chronic Pain and Sex: a Couple's Gentle Battle with Fibromyalgia." http://abcnews.go.com/Health/PainManagement/story?id=4841319&page=1.

About.com. "How to Enjoy Sexuality Despite Chronic Pain." http://seniorliving.about.com/od/sexromance/ss/chronicpainsex.htm.

Aetna InteliHealth. "Could Fibromyalgia Flare-ups Be Linked to My Menstrual Cycle?" www.intelihealth.com/IH/ihtIH/WSIHW000/24479/29516/363700.html.

Fibromyalgia Information Foundation. "Sexual Desire." http://www.myalgia.com/Treatment/connie_S.htm.

Health.com. "How People in Pain Can Revive Their Sex Lives." www.health.com/health/condition-article/0,,20189746,00.html.

Lewis & Clark College. "Maintaining Intimacy Despite Fibromyalgia." www.lclark.edu/~sherrons/topic_context.htm.

National Fibromyalgia Association. "Reclaim Your Sexuality." www
.fmaware.org/site/News2?page=NewsArticle&id=5365.

WebMD. "Fibromyalgia and Sex." www.webmd.com/fibromyalgia/guide/
fibromyalgia-and-sex.

WebMD. "Top 10 Reasons Men Don't Want Sex." http://blogs.webmd
.com/sexual-health-sex-matters/2006/09/top-10-reasons-men-dont-want
-sex.html.

WebMD. "Top 10 Reasons Women Don't Want Sex." http://blogs
.webmd.com/sexual-health-sex-matters/2006/07/top-10-reasons-women
-dont-want-sex.html.

CHAPTER 22: THE 10 BEST QUESTIONS

Before Telling Your Children About
Your Fibromyalgia

A child can ask questions that a wise man cannot answer.
—Anonymous

How do you describe fibromyalgia fatigue to an active five-year-old? How do you explain to your teenager that you're in too much pain to get out of bed today?

Your fibromyalgia can have a profound effect on your entire family. No matter what your children's ages are, telling them about "Mommy's illness" can be difficult.

This is a highly personal decision, but most child psychology experts believe that honesty is the best policy when it comes to telling children about a parent's disease. Otherwise, your illness can create an unexplained gulf between you and your children. Children tend to blame themselves for your pain in the absence of facts.

Lynne Matallana, the president of the National Fibromyalgia Association agrees, "I think it's really important that you are honest and don't cover things up. Children are very sensitive and intuitive, and any time you aren't honest or direct with them, they think things are worse than they actually are."

Maryland-based career coach Linda Pütz shares her personal story. "I've always been very open with my boys about my fibromyalgia. I always wanted them to know that if I was lying on the couch day after day, it wasn't anything that they had done."

A lot depends on the age of your children, how long you've

had your illness, and how severe your limitations are. Your children are likely to already know that there's something wrong, but a diagnosis of fibromyalgia may be the first time your symptoms have a label that you want to share with your children.

Ask *yourself* the following Best Questions as you plan out your discussion and *before* you talk with your children about your illness. There are suggestions here for both younger children and teenagers.

THE QUESTION DOCTOR SAYS:

Think of these Best Questions like a dress rehearsal for a play or big speech so you can better anticipate and relate to your special audience — your children.

You can also use these questions as a discussion guide when talking with your partner/ their father or adjust them to better fit your children's personalities or ages.

>>> THE 10 BEST QUESTIONS
Before Telling Your Children About Your Fibromyalgia

1. What is the best time and place to tell my children about my fibromyalgia?

Choose a place where you will be physically and emotionally comfortable and can avoid distractions. The best place might be your living room with the TV and cell phones off, or perhaps a favorite restaurant or park.

Seek privacy and quiet if you worry that you or your children may become emotional or distracted. Kids of all ages have notoriously short attention spans.

The most important thing is carefully choosing the setting and timing in advance rather than just launching into a discussion without first considering your needs, your children's needs, and possible outcomes of this discussion.

2. Who else (if anyone) do I want to be there when I first break the news to my children?

For example, if your children have a biological father not currently living with you, you may want to include him. Perhaps there are other close family members or friends who will support you.

If you have more than one child, think about whether or not you want to tell all your children at once or separately. If you anticipate a wide range of reactions or your children are far apart in age, telling them separately might be your best strategy.

3. What will be my children's most likely reactions to my news? How can I encourage them to talk about their feelings?

Imagine or practice this conversation before it happens. It will help you feel more prepared and self-confident for the actual discussion.

Children have a range of reactions to their moms' illnesses. They can be afraid, confused, guilty, or angry. If you have young kids, let them know that their feelings are normal and that they didn't cause your pain.

Your teen may be unpredictable, immature about bodily functions, or overly conscious of appearances. Since fibromyalgia is invisible, you may not get much sympathy or understanding from your child. Be aware that your illness may also threaten your teenager's budding independence and lead to resentments if you need his help at home.

4. What factual information about fibromyalgia do I want to give my children?

It's very important that you give your children accurate information so they don't invent their own stories. Use age-appropriate language and details to explain your symptoms. Show them books or Web sites on fibromyalgia or relate it to a time they were in pain or had the flu.

Some teens may want more facts or be ultrasensitive to wanting "the truth." Other children react by withdrawing to their own personal time and space to absorb the news and accept your illness.

As Lynne Matallana says, "Sometimes you think you have to explain all the issues, but from their perspective it's something simple like, 'Mommy, why don't you hug me anymore?'"

5. How do my symptoms impact my children's daily lives?

Stop and think for a minute about the things you can't do due to your illness. Be honest with your children that you often don't feel well. At the same time, emphasize normalcy in maintaining their daily routines.

6. How can I reassure my children?

Most kids worry about themselves when a parent is sick. Tell your children that they will be cared for no matter what even if you can't cook a four-star dinner or play ball with them like before.

Keep reassuring your children that you will do everything possible to keep their lives as normal as possible. Tell them more than once that doctors are trying to help mommy feel better again.

7. Who else can my children talk to and get support from?

Let your kids know it's okay if they want to turn to relatives, friends, religious or community leaders, teachers, coaches, or professional counselors for support, comfort, and advice. Encourage your children to ask questions of these adults for factual information and to share their feelings.

By asking yourself this question in advance, you'll have a chance to identify good sources of support. Be sensitive to your children's perspectives, too.

8. In what ways do I want my children to be involved with my care? How can they best help me? What help should I ask for?

Most child experts recommend letting your children participate in your care no matter what age they are. Give them age-appropriate tasks such as bringing you a glass of water or an extra blanket for younger children. Or let your teenager with a new driver's license drive you to doctor appointments.

On the other hand, don't demand too much of your older children. Several studies have concluded that sometimes lifelong insecurities start when a teenager is continually asked to take on household or child care chores beyond normal expectations.

9. What questions are my children likely to ask?

If you anticipate your children's questions in advance, it will give you time to prepare good answers. This preplanning step gives you more control and may ease your mind about having this talk with your kids.

Review the Best Questions in chapter 1 on initial diagnosis. Then find age-appropriate language to explain to your children what your doctor has told you.

Be prepared for your older daughter's fears about genetic risks. The evidence is currently inconclusive, but there seems to be a high prevalence of fibromyalgia in some families. A study cited in the book, *All About Fibromyalgia: A Guide for Patients and Their Families* (2002), says that about 28 percent of children of people with fibromyalgia ultimately develop the syndrome.

10. What is the worst question my children could ask me? What are their worst possible reactions? How can I be prepared for this worst-case scenario?

No matter how well prepared you are, kids are kids and are likely to surprise you with at least one off-the-wall response or question. Just don't let your runaway imagination become a justification for not telling your children at all.

Another way of thinking about this question is to consider what your children *won't* ask you. Depending on your children's ages and personalities, they may clam up, accuse you of faking it, or abruptly storm out of the room. This might be your worst-case scenario since you won't know how much they understood you or want to know.

❯ The Magic Question

What are my own most vulnerable issues, fears, and uncertainties about my fibromyalgia?

There's nothing wrong with expressing your fears and emotions to your children. But this Magic Question helps you to be flat-out honest with yourself first.

Even younger children often instinctively know where to take direct aim—either unconsciously or, with some teens, as a calculated response. For example, you may feel especially vulnerable about your diminished sex life, inability to work, or fear of more disability in the future. Working through these issues now means you'll be more self-composed and less prone to self-pity or overly emotional responses as you talk with your children. See chapter 19 on emotional health.

CONCLUSION

Don't think of this "big talk" as an all-or-nothing deal. Your children will need to hear about your illness over time. Fibromyalgia spouse and *Beyond Chaos* author Gregg Piburn advises: "We thought we were protecting our children but we learned later it's really better to be open with them."

Although fibromyalgia can be overwhelming and disruptive to your family life, you still know better than anyone else how to care for your children. By asking yourself these Best Questions in advance, you'll be better prepared to explain your illness to your children and deal with their concerns and questions.

THE 10 BEST RESOURCES

Breese, Kristine. *Cereal for Dinner: Strategies, Shortcuts, and Sanity for Moms Battling Illness.* New York: St. Martin's Griffin, 2004.

Gellman, Marc, and Debbie Tilley. *Lost and Found: A Kid's Book for Living Through Loss.* New York: HarperCollins, 1999. (Ages 9–12.)

Lewis & Clark College. "Keeping the Lines of Communication Open." www.lclark.edu/~sherrons/communication.htm.

Matallana, Lynne. "Creating a Family Plan." In *The Complete Idiot's Guide to Fibromyalgia,* 2nd ed. New York: Penguin Group, 2008.

McCue, Kathleen, and Ron Bonn, *How to Help Children Through a Parent's Serious Illness.* New York: St. Martin's Press, 1996.

National Fibromyalgia Association. "As Your Family Grows Up." www
.fmaware.org/site/News2?page=NewsArticle&id=7092.

National Fibromyalgia Association. "FM in the Family." www.fmaware
.org/site/News2?page=NewsArticle&id=7103.

National Fibromyalgia Association. "Talk Regular." www.fmaware.org/
site/News2?page=NewsArticle&id=7098.

National Fibromyalgia Association. "Will I Be a Good Parent?" www
.fmaware.org/site/News2?page=NewsArticle&id=7099.

Wallace, Daniel J., and Janice Brock Wallace. *All About Fibromyalgia: A
Guide for Patients and Their Families*. New York: Oxford University Press,
2002.

CHAPTER 23: THE 10 BEST QUESTIONS

To Decide About Telling Others

> The I in illness is isolation, and the crucial letters in wellness are we.
>
> —Anonymous

But you don't look sick!" is what people with fibromyalgia hear over and over again. Even many progressive doctors are slow to recognize fibromyalgia symptoms or misdiagnose it.

This can be a tough situation. You suffer from constant pain and fatigue yet can find only sparse sympathy from the rest of the world, sometimes even from loved ones. On the other hand, not "looking sick" gives you an interesting option to consider. Do you want other people to know about your fibromyalgia or not?

Your family and closest friends probably know. But what about your coworkers, employer, acquaintances, yoga buddies, and people in other social occasions? There's a lot of misunderstanding about fibromyalgia, so do you want to correct those misconceptions or leave them alone? Do you feel an overwhelming need to justify yourself or your fibro fog?

National Fibromyalgia Association president Lynne Matallana recalls being a healthy-looking twenty-five-year-old who needed assistance with her groceries. "Do I tell them I have a chronic pain illness or just not say anything at all? These are the daily challenges facing people with fibromyalgia."

Some people are naturally introverted and reluctant to share personal information. They worry about burdening acquaintances with their personal problems. Others are ecstatic that they finally have a named disease and splash it on their Facebook or Twitter page to educate the world about fibromyalgia.

If you are one extreme or the other—either very reserved or very open—then this chapter isn't for you because you already have clear preferences about with whom and how you'll tell about your fibromyalgia. Other people endlessly toss this dilemma around inside their heads, stressed out by internal indecision about who goes in the "Tell" bucket and who goes in the "Don't Tell" bucket. If this sounds familiar, use the following Best Questions to help resolve your indecision.

THE QUESTION DOCTOR SAYS:

This is a serious issue for some of you because your emotional and social well-being can feel threatened. Consider the people in your life who are a tremendous support to you and those who are terribly toxic or disbelieving of your illness. It's only human to want to set the record straight with these folks. You're not crazy and it's not your fault that you have fibromyalgia. Just be smart about who you "even the score" with.

⟩⟩THE 10 BEST QUESTIONS
To Decide About Telling Others

1. In the past when something bad happened to me, did I find relief and comfort in talking about it or not?

Your answer to this soul-searching question will help you understand your own needs for talking as a way to resolve issues. Think back to your previous tough situations, like a boyfriend or husband breakup, a loved one's death, nearly flunking in school, or when you lost a job promotion. What did you do? Did you talk,

talk, talk about it to anyone who would listen or share only with your most trusted confidantes? Maybe you found solace through online chats or texting to friends.

Whatever your style, just know that there's no right or wrong answer to this question. Go with the communication style that best suits you personally and not what someone else would do.

2. Who can I recruit for my "feel good" team?

Ask yourself, "Who do I know who makes me laugh, has already survived a medical crisis, or will naturally understand and comfort me?" It makes sense to confide in people who can give you something of value in return for your confidence. Find at least one good friend who will distract you with his or her sense of humor. Recruit this person to your team because laughter is great pain medicine. See chapter 26 on humor.

3. What are my motivations for telling — or not telling — certain people?

Fibromyalgia patient advocate Devin Starlanyl says, "Validation is a very important issue for some people because this is an invisible illness. We don't get the support we need because a lot of people, including physicians, think it's all in our minds."

As you sort through your motivations, in some ways it's almost like planning the guest list for your wedding. Reality hits when you wonder, "Can I really afford to feed this person?" Just like a wedding guest list, some borderline people can be moved to the "Don't Tell" bucket without consequences. Develop a flexible "telling plan" to avoid simplistic, one-size-fits-all solutions, such as "never telling" or "always being completely honest."

4. Who has a genuine need to know about my illness? Whom am I obligated to tell and when should I tell them?

There'll be obvious people to tell, such as your partner, immediate family members, and close friends. If your children are old enough, you'll feel obligated to tell them. See chapter 22.

Most likely you'll need to tell your employer, especially if you ask for extended sick leave or a flexible work schedule. And there are obvious people not to tell, like the stranger on the Denver flight or a nosy neighbor.

But most everyone else falls in between. Just make sure your "Tell" bucket isn't full of non-consequential people who have accused you of having an imaginary disease.

THE QUESTION DOCTOR SAYS:

Now it's time to switch gears and use the next five Best Questions as you go through your list of people you are contemplating telling or not. These questions will help you consider someone's specific personality characteristics and the nature of your relationship.

---

5. How will this person most likely react to my illness?

Reactions are likely to run the gamut. But just because someone is close to you doesn't mean they'll react well. Some people are constant interrupters and others are unmistakably unselfish. Once you let the cat out of the bag with your news, there's no going back.

6. Will this person make things easier or harder for me once he or she knows my news?

This is the "what's in it for me?" question. You shouldn't feel obligated to tell toxic relatives, helicopter friends, or the people least likely to understand.

Some people may surprise you with their heartfelt kindness. Others instantly morph into critics ("What did *you* do to cause this disease?), self-absorbed bubbleheads ("I'm just glad *I* don't have fibromyalgia!"), or give you the silent treatment. If someone is almost assuredly going to make you feel worse or desert you, skip telling them to minimize your own stress.

7. If I tell this person, how could it change our relationship?

This question calls for a little risk analysis. Keeping something important from a close friend or family member is more difficult than keeping a secret from the general public or acquaintances.

If you don't tell the people closest to you, they may become suspicious. Or you may find that keeping this secret has taken over your relationship and caused a gaping, unresolved distance between you.

8. Will telling this person about my fibromyalgia be an unfair burden to him or her?

Everyone has a lot going on. You may feel you don't want to bother some people or put them out. If you are worried about being a burden to others, consider:

- Most people probably do care.
- Telling someone may be easier than you initially anticipate.
- Would you be willing to help this person yourself if the tables were turned?

Just spend a minute or two in their shoes first.

9. What do I tell my employer? Am I obligated to tell?

There are many considerations here including your employer-financed health-care coverage, your need for time off, and your physical ability to continue in your current job. You may not have choices about whether or not to tell your employer, but you can probably still control how and when you tell. If in doubt about your obligations, talk with your doctor or seek other professional or legal advice.

10. How do I prefer to handle others' questions and reactions to my illness?

This is again a matter of your personal preferences for communication and whom you decide to include in your "Tell" bucket.

Even many well-intended people don't know what to say to someone in pain and may not fully understand your disease. You may need to develop a short, informative spiel that you can keep repeating to explain fibromyalgia and what is currently known about it.

Be really savvy by planning in advance how to handle people who offer to help you. Be ready with a list of simple errands or chores that won't overly burden the volunteers. For example, going to the grocery store for you or picking up your son at hockey practice can be a lifesaver.

❯ The Magic Question

Whom do I trust?

Trust is as important as it is illusive and complicated. It is a precious resource that can't be won overnight but can evaporate instantly even in the closest of relationships.

This question is potentially a deal breaker. Even the most fun, knowledgeable, convenient, important, or closest people in your life may not pass the trust test. Not sure whom to trust? Here's another Magic Question to help you decide. Ask yourself, "Would I play poker with him or her over the phone?" If you answer yes, that's real trust!

GOOD ADVICE FROM THE PRESIDENT OF THE NATIONAL FIBROMYALGIA ASSOCIATION

Lynne Matallana suggests, "Instead of saying, 'I have a chronic illness and I'm miserable,' try to get other people involved so they can better understand what it's like to have fibromyalgia.

"Use questions like, 'Have you ever had the flu? I feel like that 24/7,' or 'Have you ever pulled a muscle? That's what I feel like every day.' This person can then make a choice about how much he or she wants to know about fibromyalgia and is more likely to be empathetic to you."

CONCLUSION

No matter how well you know them, some people will surprise you by being more positive or negative than you expected. Over time, you may find this whole issue has become a nonissue.

Most important, do whatever it takes to reduce any extra stress in your life caused by your relationships. Try to forgive your friends and family members who have accused you of being crazy or misunderstand fibromyalgia. Focus your energies on those people who will be your best support system.

THE 10 BEST RESOURCES

The Fibromyalgia Experiment. "Explaining Fibromyalgia to Friends & Family." http://fibromyalgiaexperiment.com/2006/09/20/explaining -fibromyalgia-to-friends-family.

Imber-Black, Evan. *The Secret Life of Families: Making Decisions About Secrets: When Keeping Secrets Can Harm You, When Keeping Secrets Can Heal You—And How to Know the Difference.* New York: Bantam Press, 1999.

Joffe, Rosalind. "Talking About Your Chronic Illness." In *Women, Work, and Autoimmune Disease—Keep Working, Girlfriend!* New York: Demos Medical Publishing, 2008.

KeepYourSecrets.com. "Protect Your Privacy," www.keepyoursecrets.com.

National Fibromyalgia Association. "Fibromyalgia Is a Friendship Challenge—and an Opportunity." www.fmaware.org/site/News2?page= NewsArticle&id=5354.

National Fibromyalgia Association. "Fibromyalgia Support Groups." www.fmaware.org/site/PageServer?pagename=community_support GroupDirectory.

National Fibromyalgia Association. "Guidelines for Improving Communication." www.fmaware.org/site/News2?page=NewsArticle&id=6049.

Neuharth, Dan. *Secrets You Keep from Yourself: How to Stop Sabotaging Your Happiness.* New York: St. Martin's Press, 2005.

Starlanyl, Devin. "Dealing with Your World." In *Fibromyalgia Advocate.* Oakland, CA: New Harbinger Publications, 1999.

Yager, Jan. *When Friendship Hurts: How to Deal with Friends Who Betray, Abandon, or Wound You.* New York: Fireside, 2002.

CHAPTER 24: THE 10 BEST QUESTIONS

Before Joining a Support Group

Hugs Department: Always Open

—Anonymous

W hy join a support group? Because people in support groups understand; they've been there, done that, or are just learning how to cope with fibromyalgia pain or its related conditions. Where else could you find a bank vice president and a horse wrangler sharing their personal stories with each other?

A support group is defined as a group of people who meet on a regular basis with a trained group leader to discuss their concerns and feelings about the issue or disease they have in common, such as fibromyalgia, smoking, or alcoholism. There are also moderated and nonmoderated online support groups that are similar to actual meetings except the people involved rarely meet in person.

Rosie Hamlin, songwriter and singer of the 1960s hit song, "Angel Baby," says, "I would advise anyone who has fibromyalgia to join a support group, especially if you are alone. It can make the difference between losing your mind and being able to cope. If there isn't a support group in your village or town, create one."

All support groups seek to help you to restore self-confidence, connect with a community of understanding people, and learn more about fibromyalgia. People of all races and backgrounds come to support groups to find an outlet for their similar worries and issues as a result of living with this chronic illness.

You might even enjoy yourself, too. As Mark Gorkin, the self-designated "Stress Doctor," comments, "By sharing burdens with others, you can transform misery into a sense of absurdity."

The advantages to belonging to a support group include:

- Connecting with others who are going through the same thing
- Overcoming feelings of isolation, fear, and being overwhelmed
- Getting insider information on the best doctors, treatments, books, and Web sites
- Expressing confusing or frightening emotions in a safe environment
- Feeling less helpless and knowing where to get more help
- Giving loved ones touched by fibromyalgia (partner, family, and friends) an outlet

This chapter has two sets of 10 Best Questions. Ask *yourself* the first set of Best Questions to decide if a support group is right for you. If so, use the second set of Best Questions to ask *others* (the group leader or online moderator) for more information on a specific support group. This two-step process will help you determine what you really want and then help you get there.

>>> THE 10 BEST QUESTIONS
To Ask Yourself *Before Joining a Support Group*

1. Why do I want to join? What are my expectations and are they realistic?

Many people touched by fibromyalgia need a sounding board for their feelings and questions. But involvement also represents commitment, time, and energy, all which may be in short supply during flare-ups.

2. Am I a fairly open or fairly private person?

There is no right-wrong answer here. Be honest and clarify how well suited you are for a support group. Seek a one-on-one counselor if you want undivided attention, private consultations, or have major issues, like a catastrophic marriage disaster in progress.

3. Do I want an in-person group or an online group?

As you ponder this personal choice, consider your access to in-person support groups, your available time, your current state of flare-ups and pain. You might prefer 24/7 access to online chat buddies and virtual hugs. If you are a three o'clock a.m. type of person, chances are someone will be awake in Australia to reply to your online posting.

In fact, there's Dot Gerecke in rural Horsham, Australia, who says her saving grace was finding a U.S.-based online fibromyalgia group and then starting her own group Down Under. She describes her fibromyalgia correspondents as "best friends" and "close family."

4. Do I have a face-to-face support group conveniently located for me?

How you define "conveniently located" depends on your perception. *Convenient* might mean within ten miles to you while *convenient* for others is within fifty miles.

5. How comfortable will I be with this particular group?

If you aren't sure, proceed with caution and give it a fair try. Some people prefer to be with people very similar to themselves, while others aren't picky or have limited choices.

For example, Lorraine Biros, client services director of the

Mautner Project, the National Lesbian Health Organization, suggests, "It's important for some lesbian patients to find a lesbian support group if possible."

6. How emotionally rocky has my health journey been so far?

This quickie reality test will help you to assess your emotional stability and resiliency in facing down adversity and pain, and how many good listeners are already in your inner circle.

7. Realistically, will I be able to keep up with the meeting schedule and other responsibilities?

You may not have the energy if you are also working or have flare-ups. Support groups are mostly a positive experience, but if you can't keep commitments to the group it could become a new stressor.

8. Do I want my partner, other family members, or friends to accompany me to my support group meetings, join a separate support group, or not be involved at all?

Think about how much you need to discuss your partner's reactions and your other relationships. Also consider how accepting this group is of well partners. Author and fibromyalgia spouse Gregg Piburn comments, "A lot of the support groups treat the spouses as if they are invisible or mere shadows."

9. How will I feel if one of the group members becomes seriously disabled?

If you have less severe symptoms or are considerably younger than other group members, their disability may either inspire or depress you. Just consider this question before getting involved.

10. Is this going to be helpful and will I feel better each time I participate in this group?

The best support groups refuse to be falsely cheerful or overly glum. For a low-risk trial, find an online support group or one buddy to confide in before launching a public soul baring among friends and neighbors.

> The Magic Question

When I walk out of this group (or sign off from an online group), do I feel inspired to live my life more fully?

Make every moment of your life count. Your support group should be more inspiring than stressful. Chances are you already have enough of your own stress, so don't absorb anyone else's, too.

Martha Beck, well-known fibromyalgia patient, life coach, and bestselling author, offers inspiring advice, "I have such a full, active life because I never take a single second for granted."

>>> THE 10 BEST QUESTIONS
To Ask Others *Before Joining a Support Group*

1. Who leads the group? What is this person's background, formal training, and experience with people who have fibromyalgia?

A skillful and experienced group leader can make a huge difference in creating a quality experience. The ideal group leader or facilitator has been touched by fibromyalgia and has formal training in managing group dynamics.

> **THE QUESTION DOCTOR SAYS:**
>
> Find out how this group leader deals with confidentiality issues. You may be sensitive and not want your personal situation discussed outside of the support group.

2. What does the group talk about?

The best support groups share common problems, fears, knowledge, and humor. You want a sense of community and a warm atmosphere that welcomes all comers and comments with minimal criticism, judgment, whining, or self-pity parties.

3. What types of pain management issues and diagnoses do most of the participants have?

If you have choices, you may want participants with similar health challenges. For example, if you have fibromyalgia, you may or may not relate to people with different types of pain problems, such as cancer pain.

4. Are the participants either people with fibromyalgia or family members, or are both in a mixed group?

Again, this question may not matter to you or you may have limited choices. Just be aware of the different perspectives.

5. What is the size and turnover of the group?

Lively discussions happen when groups have between six and fifteen attendees. People often drift in and out of support groups, depending on their other activities and responsibilities.

If you want more long-term stability, look for a well-established group of soul mates. It will save you from having to retell your story and meet new people at each meeting.

6. Do any of the support group members socialize at times besides the regular group meetings?

You may not care about extended friendships outside of the support group. Just be aware of your own preferences ahead of time so that you don't feel either forced or neglected by the others.

7. Who is sponsoring the group and why?

Most support groups are sponsored by nonprofit groups, hospitals, medical associations, or community or religious-based organizations. Be just a little more wary of online groups until you know more about who's behind them and what, if any, hidden motives they may have, such as promoting new drugs or seeking volunteers to participate in a clinical trial.

8. Where does the group hold its meetings?

Face-to-face groups meet in hospital settings, members' homes, churches, community centers, and other public locations. The convenience of the support group's location is likely to be important to you as well as its general ambience (an impersonal hospital setting versus someone's living room).

9. Is there an online component?

There are thousands of people in online groups discussing fibromyalgia and related conditions. Some groups chat on specific issues, like treatments or side effects, while others have less direction and structure.

10. What other alternatives to face-to-face support group meetings do I have?

You may need help beyond a support group's capability. If so, seek private counseling with a therapist, social worker, or trusted religious or community leader. See chapters 19 and 20 on emotions and partner relationships.

❭ The Magic Question

How does the group leader protect participants' emotions and egos during group discussions?

There are certain risks to being an active member of a support group and sharing your true thoughts and feelings. A first-class group facilitator creates a safe place for people to share their stories and personal vulnerabilities.

The use of ground rules for discussion, such as, "All comments are welcome, but no personal attacks," defines the boundaries of acceptable discussion topics and behaviors and creates a safety net for all participants.

Dr. Patrick Wood, a fibromyalgia expert in Seattle, adds, "Look for a support group with a healthy mindset, one that's pro-active and pro-health rather than encouraging people who have their identities wrapped up in being sick to do a lot of complaining. A group where people who want to 'out-do each other' in 'who is the most disabled one here' needs to be redirected by a good moderator to a more healthy discussion."

CONCLUSION

Seeking a support group may be the healthiest thing you can do for yourself, even if you usually aren't a "group person" or can think of a million excuses. Just talking with others who understand your symptoms and know you aren't crazy can be a huge relief. Support groups are also a great way to learn the latest on fibromyalgia treatments and share fibro-friendly doctors' names.

And support groups aren't just for fibromyalgia only. Perhaps you are trying to improve your well-being in other ways. For example, the American Lung Association's national program manager for smoking cessation, Bill Blatt, suggests, "You'll be with other people who are going through exactly the same thing and they can offer advice and help you be successful."

THE 10 BEST RESOURCES

American Chronic Pain Association. "Groups." http://theacpa.org/about/groups.asp.

FibroAction. "Support Groups—UK." www.fibroaction.org/Pages/Support-Groups.aspx.

FibroDoc's. "Welcome You!" www.fibrodoc.org.

Fibrohugs. "Welcome." www.fibrohugs.org.

The Fibromyalgia Community. "Online Discussion Groups." www.fmscommunity.org/online.htm.

MDJunction. "Fibromyalgia Support Group." http://www.mdjunction.com/fibromyalgia.

National Fibromyalgia Association. "Network of Support Groups by State." www.fmaware.org/site/PageServer?pagename=community_supportGroupDirectory.

National Fibromyalgia Association. "Support Group Information." www.fmaware.org/site/PageServer?pagename=community_supportGroupInformation.

WebMD. "Fibromyalgia Support Group." http://boards.webmd.com/webx?14@@.5987f42a.

Yahoo! "Browse Groups about Fibromyalgia." http://health.dir.groups.yahoo.com/dir/1600061682.

CHAPTER 25: THE 10 BEST QUESTIONS

For Financial Health After Fibromyalgia

We all need money, but there are degrees of desperation.
—Anthony Burgess

A s a person with fibromyalgia, you may face financial challenges as a result of your illness. Chronic disease not only affects your health but also your wallet. According to the National Institutes of Health, pain costs the U.S. economy more than $100 billion annually in health care and lost productivity.

Everyone's situation is different. Perhaps you've been the main breadwinner in your family and now you are contemplating disability leave. Maybe you are ready to retire anyway, have other income, or need a job that doesn't require standing up for long intervals.

Health Day News for Healthier Living reports that 79 million Americans said they had trouble paying off their medical bills and debts in 2007. If this sounds familiar, your financial difficulties won't be solved easily. But having a heart-to-heart talk with yourself is a great first step. Think of your health troubles as a wake-up call to get more financially savvy.

Keep in mind that if you have severe fibro fog, you need to make financial decisions with a clear head. The following Best Questions and tips should not be used as a substitute for professional financial or tax advice.

>>> THE 10 BEST QUESTIONS
For Financial Health After Fibromyalgia

1. How well organized are my/our personal financial papers, accounts, and records?

Managing financial records and bills is a challenge for most people. You may resist the tedious task of creating boring filing systems. But careful financial planning starts with putting financial documents in one place and taming any "clutter monsters" lurking under your bed.

Important financial and legal documents include:

- Bank and brokerage account information
- Birth certificates
- Deeds, mortgage papers, and ownership statements
- Passwords, account numbers, and safe-deposit access
- Insurance policies
- Monthly or outstanding bills
- Pension and other retirement benefit summaries
- Rental income paperwork
- College scholarship and grant money forms for your children
- Social security information
- Stock and bond certificates

2. What are my/our financial assets?

A **financial asset** is anything you own that has monetary value. Financial assets generally refer to paper assets like accounts and funds as well as tangible property, including house ownership and the vehicles sitting in your driveway.

When you are writing down all your assets, don't forget these:

- Home and real estate holdings
- 401(k) accounts
- IRAs
- Mutual funds
- Stocks and bonds
- Employee stock options
- College savings
- Other savings
- Insurance policies
- Cash
- Cars, trucks, boats, and motorcycles
- Other valuables, such as appraised collectibles, antiques, and personal property

3. What are my/our debts and expenses?

Creating and living within a budget is a necessary evil. Norman Berk, a certified financial planner in Birmingham, Alabama, comments, "A budget can help keep you out of debt as well as provide for a means to reduce existing debt. It also can be the focal point for serious review of expenditures so a plan can be developed to have the extra funds if they are suddenly necessary."

Start by identifying how you've spent your money in the past. Your debts may already be under control, but chances are they are less than ideal. Be aware that unexpected medical bills are one of the most common causes of personal bankruptcies.

Include the following debts and expenses on your list:

- Mortgage payment or rent
- Credit card payments
- Auto loans
- Personal loans
- Child care expenses or child-support payments
- Insurance costs
- Living expenses including food, clothing, utilities, fuel, transportation, parking, cable and Internet charges, personal care, routine doctor and dentist bills, drugs, entertainment, holiday gifts, vacations, hobbies, home repair, taxes, school tuition, magazine/newspaper subscriptions, and other miscellaneous costs

Get your FICO score if you don't already know it. A FICO score is based on your credit history and is widely used to determine if you are a good credit risk. FICO scores (an acronym for the Fair Isaac Corporation at www.myfico.com) range from a low of 300 to a perfect 850 score.

Don't go nuts over this exercise, but don't skip it either. The more you understand your current financial status, the better prepared you'll be for new or ongoing medical bills.

4. What is my/our health insurance coverage for treatments and other medical bills related to this diagnosis?

A long, protracted search for a correct fibromyalgia diagnosis and then ongoing medical bills can be costly. If you are covered through your employer, get a copy of your policy and familiarize yourself with your coverage's details. If fibromyalgia is not covered, check to see if some related symptoms are, like sleep disorders or irritable bowel syndrome. Take insurance cards to all appointments.

Lynne Matallana, president of the National Fibromyalgia Association, advises, "Make sure your insurance company covers your fibromyalgia before you buy a policy. It might be listed as an exclusionary illness. It's a real catch-22. If you have fibromyalgia the insurance company may not cover your life insurance, but when you say that fibromyalgia is a real illness, your health insurance won't cover you for it either."

Sidestep costly surprises. Don't end up in insurance limbo land or the poorhouse.

5. Do I want to be off from work or am I able (and happier) to continue working? How many days can I afford to be out?

Consider your options. Some people devote their full-time energies to healing and avoiding their stressful workplaces, while others relish work as a welcome distraction from their health problems. Some people with fibromyalgia who have major flare-ups or battle severe fibro fog are not able to work. Still others find a job they can do from home, work part time, or retire.

Your need to keep an income may drive all else. You may be compelled to work in order to pay medical bills and other looming debts.

The Family and Medical Leave Act allows most workers in the United States twelve weeks of leave each year for a serious illness. You don't necessarily have to take all your leave at once.

6. Do I/we have a designated financial power of attorney? Do I/we have a medical power of attorney? Do I/we have a legally binding document stating who this person is?

Taking care of this business is hard. But think of these legal protections as an act of generosity and kindness for your loved ones.

You are relieving them of the burden of making difficult decisions later.

According to Chicago-based certified financial planner Cicily Carson Maton, "A power of attorney for health is very important to have in place so your agent can pay your bills and take care of your affairs. It is absolutely vital."

A **medical power of attorney** is a separate but similar document that specifies your wishes if you become medically incapacitated. Consider getting this document prepared before any surgeries or long-distance travel for treatments. Your hospital or clinic may provide this form for free, but check with a lawyer or financial planner for a final blessing.

7. Do I/we have an estate plan, a will, and a living will? Are my/our other legal affairs in order?

Estate planning is the orderly process of preparing to transfer your affairs and assets to your intended beneficiaries. A good estate plan should also minimize taxes, court costs, and attorneys' fees, while addressing your welfare and needs. Most adults need an estate plan regardless of the size of their estate.

A **will** is not just for rich people. No matter how much you have, a will helps to ensure that your children and other beneficiaries will not suffer undue confusion or anxiety about your wishes.

A **living will** (also called a **living trust** or **medical directive**) gives you the opportunity to declare your intentions about lifesaving efforts on your behalf and to appoint a representative to ensure your intentions are followed.

8. What are my/our insurance options?

Look at all your insurance options, including health-care coverage, Medicare, disability, long-term care, veterans' benefits, and life insurance plans. Understanding these policies now can save you time and money later.

9. What are my/our options and eligibility for government assistance programs or other assistance in paying medical bills? What leave, medical benefits, and schedule flexibility can I reasonably expect from my employer?

The primary government health-care program for people over sixty-five is Medicare. Other government assistance programs include:

- Social Security Disability Income (SSDI)
- Supplemental Security Income (SSI). See www.ssa.gov/dibplan/dqualify5.htm
- Veterans' benefits. See www.vba.va.gov/VBA
- Tax deductions and credits
- Care credit

SSDI is for workers under age sixty-five who can prove an inability to work. SSI guarantees a monthly income for people age sixty-five or older, disabled, and with limited income.

Medicaid pays for medical care for very low income people with no other resources. Veterans may qualify for health and long-term care benefits. There are also various tax and care credits available. Check with www.benefitscheckup.org and the financial assistance organizations listed in the resource sections of this book. See www.socialsecurity.gov for more information.

10. Do I/we need help from a professional financial advisor?

Investigate services and costs before answering this question. Look for a certified financial planner with proven experience in dealing with chronically ill people.

As you are calling around, ask for the advisors' specific services; if they sell products (be wary); their personal philosophy on financial planning (conservative, aggressive, etc.); who exactly you'll be working with; if charges are by the hour, flat fees, or commissions; and a written list of services and charges.

Paul Yurachek, a certified financial planner with Ameriprise Financial Services, says, "When people are aging, it creates a whole new set of issues, especially if there's a spouse involved. As financial advisors, we try to alleviate their concerns about money."

Financial planner Cicily Carson Maton advises, "If you didn't have any financial planning in place or have a financial advisor prior to your diagnosis, reach out to those people around you that you trust and ask for their help."

❯ The Magic Question

How can I/we avoid letting fibromyalgia ruin my/our financial health?

This question is aimed at another potential threat to your financial stability—you.

You do have some control. Find ways to cut back on expenses and clarify your priorities. Look at your spending habits as honestly as possible.

Here are some red flags from the National Foundation for Credit Counseling for poor money management:

- Always late with bill payments
- Withdrawn funds from retirement or savings accounts to pay current expenses
- Calls from creditors about overdue bills
- Credit card cash advances to pay off other creditors
- Minimum repayments on installment charges
- Overtime work to make ends meet

CONCLUSION

No matter what your financial, insurance, and employment circumstances are, you can deal with them more proactively if you take the time now to assess your situation and figure out how to locate financial assistance if needed.

When that's done, you can really focus your energies on being pain free and healthy. You won't be trying to fight financial fatigue and insurance exhaustion at the same time you are coping with fibromyalgia pain and fatigue.

THE 10 BEST RESOURCES

American Pain Foundation. "Financial Information & Assistance Articles & Web Links." www.painfoundation.org/page.asp?file=Links/Financial.htm.

HealthWell Foundation, "Helping Patients Afford the Medical Treatments They Need." HealthWell Foundation, www.healthwellfoundation.org/index.aspx.

H.E.L.P. "Financial Issues." www.help4srs.org/finance/finintro.htm.

Medicare. "State Health Insurance Assistance Program." www.medicare.gov/contacts/static/allStateContacts.asp.

National Council on Aging. "Benefits Checkup." (Searchable program.) www.benefitscheckup.org.

National Fibromyalgia Association. "A Few Financial Planning Questions for People with Fibromyalgia." www.fmaware.org/site/News2?page =NewsArticle&id=5282.

Patient Access Network Foundation. "How to Apply." www.patient accessnetwork.org/HowApply.html.

Patient Advocate Foundation. "Resources for Solving Insurance and Healthcare Access Problems." www.patientadvocate.org.

PPARx. "Partnership for Prescription Assistance." https://www.pparx .org/Intro.php.

Social Security Administration. "Online Social Security Handbook." www.ssa.gov/OP_Home/handbook/ssa-hbk.htm.

CHAPTER 26: THE 10 *WORST* QUESTIONS
To Ask Someone with Fibromyalgia

Laughter is an instant vacation.

—Milton Berle

Living with fibromyalgia is good reason to feel sad, stressed, and depressed sometimes. You are not crazy. You are not lazy. And you really do have a real disease called fibromyalgia. But sometimes it seems that you just "can't get no respect."

One way to cope is to let a good sense of humor be your best friend. Humor can be a powerful ally. Over the past decades, studies have found that humor can reduce physical pain and stress. The message is simple: Humor is healing. The medicinal power of laughter can fight your symptoms and lighten your load.

Patty Wooten is a nurse in Santa Cruz, California, who specializes in the therapeutic benefits of humor. She says, "Humor and laughter change our emotional state. For the moments of laughter, there are feelings of delight and joy, so we break the negative cycle. The other powerful thing about humor is that once you start to laugh, you feel more in control."

In his pioneering 1979 book, *Anatomy of an Illness,* Norman Cousins says "laughter therapy" cured him from a supposedly irreversible disease. Cousins discovered while watching old Marx Brothers films and television's *Candid Camera* shows that ten minutes of belly laughs helped him sleep pain free for two hours.

Welcome to the Hall of Shame, the Worst Questions asked by well-meaning but clueless people about your fibromyalgia. These awful questions come from people who don't know what else to say or are totally insensitive, and were compiled from fibromyalgia online discussion groups, patients, and other sources. Here's what *not* to ask a person with fibromyalgia.

THE QUESTION DOCTOR SAYS:

How well does your sense of humor protect you from disease? Find out by taking the humor questionnaire by cardiologist Dr. Michael Miller at the University of Maryland Medical Center. Go to www.umm.edu/news/releases/humor_survey.htm.

〉〉〉THE 10 *WORST* QUESTIONS
To Ask Someone with Fibromyalgia

1. You don't look sick. How do I know you're not just faking it?

This common question is so insensitive! How many times have you heard it yourself? What does it take for some sympathy and understanding—lots of gushing blood and broken bones?

2. Are you just trying to get out of work?

Asked by a suspicious or even jealous coworker, she wonders if you are secretly avoiding a demanding project or have ulterior motives so you can work from home.

3. Did I tell you about my awful headache last week?

One of the most universally despised and most common "Worst Questions" involves telling a long shaggy dog story about someone else's experience with pain. Most people mean well, but they end up hijacking your conversation and have no idea what your level of pain is like.

4. What did you do to get fibromyalgia?

This questioner has assumed that somehow you are to blame for your own illness or it is contagious. Just look him in the eye and say, "No one knows for sure what causes fibromyalgia. I didn't cause it. I just got lucky."

5. How does it feel to be losing your mind?

Many people with fibro fog like to make jokes about it because it's often embarrassing or scary. Fight this lousy Worst Question with a witty comeback like, "Yeah, I'm out of my mind, but I'll be back in five minutes."

6. Are you sure you don't have Alzheimer's disease instead of this fibro fog stuff?

No, how about you? Remember that half the people you know (including the creep who asked this question) are below average on IQ tests. Did he ever stop to think and forget to start again? Or maybe his IQ test results were negative numbers.

7. Since you're disabled, can I borrow your handicap parking pass?

Some people are rude, stupid, or insensitive—or all three! Oh yes, and act illegally, too.

8. Can you still have sex?

Ditto, with an emphasis on rude. Coming from the right person, this can be a kind and caring question. But if asked in a prying manner or by someone you aren't close to, it becomes an out-of-bounds question. The asker most likely really wants to know, "What's going on in your bedroom and personal life?"

9. Should you be doing that?

Coming from the right person with the right tone of voice this question shows concern for your health. But if your overbearing father-in-law who just ran the Marine Marathon in record time asks you, chances are you have a self-appointed health freak looking over your shoulder and threatening your independence.

10. How long do you have to live?

This Worst Question may come from the person's ignorance that the words *chronic* and *terminal* mean different things. You can happily inform her that you have no plans for going anywhere soon.

❯ The Magic Question

What's for dinner?

Sigh. Sob. Scream. Laugh. Reply, "Takeout again, my dear."

CONCLUSION

Maybe you've heard even Worse Questions than these. If so, don't hesitate to share them with your friends. Living with chronic pain is no laughing matter, but even in the worst of times a good belly laugh can do wonders.

THE 10 BEST RESOURCES

Allen Klein.com. "Humor and Healing—Related Links." www.allen klein.com/links.htm.

Association for Applied and Therapeutic Humor. "AATH e-zine." www .aath.org/ezine/ezine-2008_02.html.

Buckman, Elcha. *The Handbook of Humor: Clinical Applications in Psychotherapy.* Malabar, FL: Krieger Publishing, 1994.

Halpern, Susan P. *The Etiquette of Illness: What to Say When You Can't Find the Words.* New York: Bloomsbury, 2004.

The Humor Project, Inc. "Humor Sourcebook." www.humorproject.com/publications/sourcebook.pdf.

Jest for the Health of It! "Resources/Articles." www.jesthealth.com.

Klein, Allen. *The Courage to Laugh.* New York: Tarcher/Putnam Books, 1998.

Neuharth, Dan. *Secrets You Keep from Yourself: How to Stop Sabotaging Your Happiness.* New York: St. Martin's Griffin, 2005.

Suite101.com. "Fibromyalgia: Those Stinging Comments Made by Others." www.suite101.com/article.cfm/fibromyalgia/11290.

Wooten, Patty. *Compassionate Laughter: Jest for Your Health,* 2nd. ed. Santa Cruz, CA: Jest Press. 2002.

CHAPTER 27: THE 10 BEST QUESTIONS
For Your Spiritual Health and
Fibromyalgia

Do not be afraid of tomorrow, for God is already there.

—Anonymous

Having a chronic, painful disease with no known cure ignites a spiritual crisis for many people with fibromyalgia. Some people find their belief in God shaken to the core. Others find deeper meaning in their chosen faith.

Spirituality is defined here as a general awareness of a force greater than the individual self. Religion is only one aspect of spirituality. In this holistic definition, spirituality can also mean connecting with nature, holding unspoken beliefs, or finding peace of mind in the back row of a yoga class. Dr. Christina Puchalski, the director of George Washington University's Institute for Spirituality and Health, defines spirituality as "that part of us which gives us the ultimate meaning in life." A "faith community" is used here to broadly mean any group of people who share the same beliefs.

While there is no proof that spirituality or prayers can cure disease, many studies have shown the importance of faith in healing. Prayer can reduce your stress, anxiety, and depression, promote a more positive outlook, and strengthen your will to live despite the pain.

Martha Beck, well-known fibromyalgia patient, life coach, and bestselling author, offers this positive advice. "In the world of psychology and spirituality, everything is made from its opposite. If a disease is disempowering, then its opposite is the most power you can possibly pick up in your own life. Fibromyalgia challenges you to become empowered at a level that is far greater than you might ever consider if you hadn't had the disease."

A ten-year study by the U.S. Office of Technology Assessment found an 83 percent positive effect on physical health. Another set of studies measuring spirituality's benefits concluded that 92 percent of the patients reported positive benefits.

As Dr. Christina Puchalski observes, "Healing is more than just a cure. It's how people see themselves. You can see yourself as broken or you can see yourself as a whole person who is not succumbing to this illness." Dr. Patrick Wood, director of the Fibromyalgia Care Center agrees, "Prayer and mediation used properly have a role in stress reduction and pain management."

Ask yourself the following Best Questions as you explore your own spiritual journey as a person with fibromyalgia. Dr. Hamilton Beazley, scholar and author of the book *No Regrets,* believes, "Best Questions are like a set of physical exercises to keep the body in tune, except these questions keep us spiritually healthy."

THE QUESTION DOCTOR SAYS:

Pace yourself as you ask yourself these Best Questions. In order to reflect fully on each question, you may prefer to ponder them over the course of a few days, weeks, or months. Perhaps one question per day will work for you.

Ask your own Best Questions as well. You may also choose to discuss these questions with your loved ones or your faith community.

〉〉〉THE 10 BEST QUESTIONS
For Your Spiritual Health and Fibromyalgia

1. How important is spiritual faith or religion in my life?

A major diagnosis often results in a reassessment of the importance of your spiritual life. Some people may deny their faith and
question how God could let something this bad happen to them.
They may develop private doubts, skepticism, cynicism, or a sense
of hollowness. For others, this disease translates into a reaffirma-
tion of their faith in a new or deeper way.

Dr. Christina Puchalski comments, "Fibromyalgia may not be
life threatening, but it is lifestyle threatening. Pain is very difficult to live with. Where spirituality comes into play, is in the acceptance of pain. Illness is a spiritual journey."

No matter what your previous connection has been to your
faith, you may instantly know your answer to this question or you
may need to ponder it long and hard. Either way, it's your starting
point for considering your spiritual health.

2. Am I angry at God because I have fibromyalgia? If so, how can I make peace with Him?

People who have actively practiced their religious faith, regularly
attended religious services, and tried to be a "good" person may
feel a terrible sense of unfairness. You may lash out and ask, "Why
are You punishing me?" "What kind of God are you?"

Dr. Hamilton Beazley says, "Sometimes you have to forgive
God. The anger ties you to the past. It means you aren't free." If
you can't get beyond the hurt or anger, seek professional counseling so that your emotions won't cripple your daily life.

Albert Einstein once said, "God may be subtle, but He isn't
plain mean."

3. What role do I want my faith or religious beliefs to play in my battle against fibromyalgia?

People have used prayer and other spiritual practices for thousands of years as tools for healing. A 2004 study by the National Center for Complementary and Alternative Medicine found that 45 percent of the people surveyed have used prayer to relieve symptoms of their illness. Dr. Brent A. Bauer, director of Mayo Clinic's Complementary and Integrative Medicine, advises, "Recognizing the spiritual component of our wellness is a critical component."

Your faith may be a source of strength and comfort, may serve as a guiding force for making tough decisions, or may serve as a light at the end of the tunnel called "uncertainty." Some estranged couples or families touched by chronic illness find that their shared faith keeps their communication lifeline open during tough times.

4. What support did I find in the past from my faith community?

Many people describe themselves as spiritual but don't participate in any formal religious institution or rituals. Whether your faith is connected to Christianity, Judaism, Buddhism, Islam, or Mother Nature, consider how much you have experienced comfort from your past associations with other people in your faith community.

What has been the nature of your prayers in the past? How did you respond to the past challenges in your life when you turned to your faith for comfort and hope? Who and what helped you the most?

5. How can I reconnect with my faith community to find new meaning?

A Gallup Poll in 2001 found that 43 percent of Americans attended religious services at least once a week. Sometimes people's childhood religious affiliations slip away or are consciously abandoned in adulthood. A fibromyalgia diagnosis may awaken your need to be part of the faith community of your choice again or perhaps to reassess your religious roots.

Martha Beck shares her personal story as an example. "My religion made my body hurt. It wasn't a real option for me to keep trying to pretend that I was a good Mormon girl because I was in a lot of pain when I pretended that way. Part of my own spiritual journey was to leave the religion of my childhood."

In addition to offering a close-knit and supportive environment, some faith communities host discussion groups or provide financial support. Maryland-based career and life coach, Linda Pütz, describes her own odyssey with chronic pain. "My faith and finding a good faith community have sustained me. I can go, learn, and be surrounded by others who are thinking about kindness, mercy, and love instead of politics, finances, or long commutes."

6. How much do I want to share my spirituality or religious beliefs with my loved ones?

Some people believe their spirituality is a private affair and choose not to share it with even their closest loved ones. Others wouldn't dream of excluding their loved ones from their beliefs and active religious observances.

Part of this deeper quest is deciding how much of your spirituality and religious beliefs you want to be public and how much you want to be private.

7. How can my faith or religious beliefs give me the additional strength and courage that I need right now?

This may seem like your darkest hour. Chances are you are facing a newly redefined life that includes many lifestyle and medical challenges that may seem daunting right now. You may see your faith or religion as your "rock of Gibraltar," a steadfast light to guide you and your loved ones during the future uncertainties and changes ahead for you.

Dr. Herbert Benson, mind-body pioneer and author of the classic book *The Relaxation Response*, says, "Frequently a person will choose a prayer to repeat as a way to quiet the mind and as an automatic linkage to spirituality. When people evoke the Relaxation Response, even using secular terms, they feel more spiritual. This is called the 'Faith Factor.'"

8. What would Jesus (or another role model) do if He had fibromyalgia?

Thinking of a role model, either a great spiritual teacher like Jesus, Buddha, or Muhammad, or a sweet spiritual person in your life, like a favorite rabbi, aunt, or former priest, is like having a mentor on call. Ask yourself what this person would do in your situation.

This isn't to suggest that you are "channeling" the spirits or some other hocus-pocus, but rather you are tapping into the wisdom that knowing this person has given you. Let that other person's strength be your anchor and companion.

Your spiritual guide can be a trusted family member or other loved one. As Dr. Christina Puchalski says, "What people are really looking for is someone who can just be with them without trying to fix their problem, just help them get through this time."

9. What lessons does God want me to learn from my pain?

Chronic pain may lead you to search for new meaning. You may feel compelled to ask the ultimate biggest and Best Questions of life, "Who am I?" "Why am I here?" "What does my life mean?"

Most of us rarely acknowledge our mortality. But living with pain every day means you may be now ready to strengthen your relationship with God.

Perhaps His lessons for you will be profound or involve new joy in simple daily pleasures. Whatever your lessons, asking this Best Question will help you on the path of accepting your disease.

For example, Linda Pütz recalls how a major fibromyalgia flare-up that coincided with the events of September 11, 2001, had a silver lining. "I felt terrible about only being able to open a can of soup for everyone's dinner. But on balance, I was more present and a better listener for my five- and nine-year-old boys and the neighborhood boys who shared popcorn and their nightmares with each other on my front stoop. I would have been too busy if it hadn't been for my illness. I remember hurting all over, like having the flu, but being so riveted by their openness that I was carried out of myself and simply focused on them, a real blessing."

10. Do I want my doctors to address faith issues during my health care? If so, what are my expectations?

This may not be an option if your doctors favor a clinical approach to care. Not all doctors have soft sides or open personalities. And perhaps you would be uncomfortable talking with them about faith or don't have enough time during office visits.

Dr. Betty Ferrell, RN, a clinician and research scientist in pain management at City of Hope National Medical Center in Duarte, California, believes, "Pain has a spiritual and existential dimension and to ignore that is to damage the essence of the patient."

Some people with fibromyalgia discover an overlooked opportunity to connect with their doctors in a deeper way than previously imagined. The key is clarifying your own expectations in advance about what role, if any, your doctor has here.

❯ The Magic Question

What unmet needs do I have concerning my faith or spirituality?

Regardless of how frequently you practice your faith or pray, you may benefit from coming to grips now with any past regrets or missed opportunities that have bothered you. For example, there may be a faith-based ritual, such as a baptism or church-blessed wedding, which you feel is overdue. Perhaps your diagnosis will prompt you to reach out to a long-estranged parent, sibling, son, or old friend.

Living well with fibromyalgia can mean finding a true reordering of your life's priorities. Spiritual healing can be a powerful component in your journey to better health and quality of life.

CONCLUSION

"Ask and it will be given to you; seek and you will find; knock and the door will be opened to you. For everyone who asks receives; he who seeks finds; and to him who knocks, the door will be opened." (Matthew 7:7–8)

THE 10 BEST RESOURCES

American Academy of Family Physicians. "Spirituality and Health." http://familydoctor.org/online/famdocen/home/articles/650.html.

Beazley, Hamilton. *No Regrets: A Ten-Step Program for Living in the Present and Leaving the Past Behind.* Hoboken, NJ: John Wiley & Sons, 2004.

George Washington University Institute for Spirituality and Health. "The Role of Spirituality in Health and Illness." www.gwish.org.

National Fibromyalgia Association. "Spirituality." www.fmaware.org/site/PageServer?pagename=topics_spirituality.

Open Directory Project. "Religion and Spirituality." www.dmoz.org/Society/Religion_and_Spirituality.

Spiritual Experiences. "Spiritual Experiences and Spirituality." www.spiritual-experiences.com.

Tolle, Eckhart. *A New Earth: Awakening to Your Life's Purpose.* New York: Penguin, 2008.

University of Minnesota's Center for Spirituality & Healing. "Home Page." www.csh.umn.edu.

Warren, Rick. *The Purpose Driven® Life: What on Earth Am I Here For?* Grand Rapids, MI.: Zondervan Press, 2007.

Wikipedia. "Spirituality." http://en.wikipedia.org/wiki/Spirituality.

CONCLUSION:

Living Well with Fibromyalgia

You, interrupted. That's what happens when you develop a chronic illness like fibromyalgia. It changes your life forever.

The good news is that research at this very moment will soon help people with fibromyalgia. Dr. Daniel Clauw, a fibromyalgia expert and professor at the University of Michigan, says, "The level of knowledge regarding fibromyalgia is improving dramatically. If you're a patient, hang in there because help is on the way." Seattle-based fibromyalgia expert Dr. Patrick Wood agrees, "This is an interesting moment in fibromyalgia history. Fibromyalgia is finally coming into its own. It's expanding weekly. It's very much an evolving science."

The main focus of this book has been *you*. As Harvard University's Dr. Daniel Forman says, "The real heroes of this story are the patients and what they do every day to organize their lives in a healthier way."

Martha Beck says, "I tell people who have fibromyalgia, 'Congratulations. You were born with an extra-sensitive and powerful compass. Your fabulous, extraordinarily sensitive and accurate compass is giving you a signal that you need to pay attention to. It gives meaning to your pain. Even your worst experience transforms your path into a gift.'"

The president of the National Fibromyalgia Association and a longtime sufferer, Lynne Matallana, advises, "It's really important for people with fibromyalgia to understand that how well you communicate and how honest and direct you are by asking questions is going to help you to cope better with your fibromyalgia. If you refuse to open the dialogue, it's going to hurt you personally."

Think of this book as the start of a lifetime of asking your own Best Questions about everything. Questions are for smarties, not dummies. It's not what you know. It's what you *ask* that really matters.

Knowledge truly is power. Asking Best Questions is your secret weapon to being an empowered patient who is actively involved in your own health care and a team player with your doctors.

Dot Gerecke in Horsham, Australia, who has suffered with fibromyalgia since 1982, proclaims, "You are not a victim. You are a survivor and you have a life!"

Remember that a good mind knows the right answers, but a great mind knows the right questions. Now it's your turn. You are not just living with fibromyalgia, you are actually thriving with it.

Resources

We regret any errors or omissions on this resource list. Inclusion on this list does not imply endorsement by the publisher or the author. We defined "best resource" as the most practical and content-rich information available with an emphasis on question lists and free online access.

THE 10 VERY BEST RESOURCES

Fibromyalgia Network. "Home page." www.fmnetnews.com.

Matallana, Lynne, and Laurence A. Bradley. *The Complete Idiot's Guide to Fibromyalgia,* 2nd ed. New York: Penguin Group, 2009.

Mayo Clinic. "Fibromyalgia." www.mayoclinic.com/health/fibromyalgia/DS00079.

MedicineNet. "Fibromyalgia." www.medicinenet.com/fibromyalgia/article.htm.

MedlinePlus. "Fibromyalgia." www.nlm.nih.gov/medlineplus/fibromyalgia.html.

National Fibromyalgia Association. "Fibromyalgia Topics A-Z." www.fmaware .org/site/PageServer?pagename=topics.

National Fibromyalgia Research Association. "Welcome!" www.nfra.net.

PubMed. "Search." www.ncbi.nlm.nih.gov/sites/entrez.

St. Amand, R. Paul, and Claudia Craig Marek. *What Your Doctor May Not Tell You About Fibromyalgia: The Revolutionary Treatment That Can Reverse the Disease.* New York: Wellness Central, 2006.

Starlanyl, Devin J., and Mary Ellen Copeland. *Fibromyalgia and Chronic Myofascial Pain: A Survival Manual,* 2nd ed., Oakland, Calif.: New Harbinger Publications, 2001.

CHAPTER RESOURCES

Chapter 1 — The 10 Best Questions About Your Diagnosis of Fibromyalgia

American Pain Association. "APF Pain Resource Locator." www.painfoundation .org/ResourceLocator.asp.

Berne, Katrina, Robert M. Bennett, and Daniel L. Peterson. *Chronic Fatigue*

Syndrome, Fibromyalgia, and Other Invisible Illnesses. Alameda, CA: Hunter House, 2002.

Centers for Disease Control and Prevention. "Fibromyalgia." www.cdc.gov/arthritis/arthritis/fibromyalgia.htm.

FibroCenter. "Causes of Fibromyalgia." www.fibrocenter.com/images/FM_Causes.pdf.

Fibromyalgia Association UK. "Welcome." www.fibromyalgia-associationuk.org/index.php.

FM-CFS Canada. "Educational Resources for Patients." www.fm-cfs.ca/resources.html.

Kelly, Julie W., and Rosalie Devonshire. *Taking Charge of Fibromyalgia: Everything You Need to Know to Manage Fibromyalgia,* 6th ed. Minneapolis: Fibromyalgia Educational Systems, 2008.

Pellegrino, Mark J., and David Schumick. *Inside Fibromyalgia with Mark J. Pellegrino, MD.* Columbus, OH: Anadem Publishing, 2001.

Staud, Roland, and Christine Adamec. *Fibromyalgia for Dummies.* New York: Wiley Publishing, 2007.

Wallace, Daniel J., and Daniel J. Clauw. *Fibromyalgia and Other Central Pain Syndromes.* Philadelphia: Lippincott, Williams & Wilkins, 2005.

Wikipedia. "Fibromyalgia." http://en.wikipedia.org/wiki/Fibromyalgia.

Chapter 2 — The 10 Best Questions to Get a Reliable Referral for the Best Doctor

American Medical Association. "AMA ePhysician Profiles." www.ama-assn.org/ama/pub/category/2672.html.

Boston Central. "Doctor Referrals." www.bostoncentral.com/healthcare/doctor_ref.php.

Consumers' Checkbook. "Top Doctors." www.checkbook.org/doctors/pageone.cfm. (Subscription required.)

Dowie, Jack, and Arthur Elstein. *Professional Judgment: A Reader in Clinical Decision Making.* Cambridge: Cambridge University Press, 1988.

MedicineNet. "How to Choose a Doctor." www.medicinenet.com/script/main/art.asp?articlekey=47649.

Chapter 3 — The 10 Best Questions for Choosing a Best Doctor

American Board of Medical Specialties. "Bedside Manner, Board Certification Matter." www.abms.org/News_and_Events/Media_Newsroom/Releases/release_ABMS_C onsumer_Survey.aspx.

American Board of Medical Specialties. "How to Be a Smart Patient." www.abms
.org/Who_We_Help/Consumers/educate.aspx.

The American Board of Psychiatry and Neurology. "Initial Certification in the Subspecialty of Pain Medicine." www.abpn.com/pain.htm.

American Psychological Association. "Find a Psychologist." http://locator.apa .org.

Federation of State Medical Boards. "Welcome to DocInfo." www.docinfo.org.

FibroCenter. "Finding a Health Care Professional." www.fibrocenter.com/content/ finding_hcp_tools_and_resources.jsp.

Leeds, Dorothy. *Smart Questions to Ask Your Doctor.* New York: Harper Paperbacks, 1992.

National Fibromyalgia Association. "The Perfect Fit." www.fmaware.org/site/ News2?page=NewsArticle&id=5728.

National Medical Association. "Physician Locator." (For African-Americans.) www.nmanet.org.

WebMD. "WebMD Physician Directory." http://doctor.webmd.com/physician_ finder/home.aspx?sponsor=core.

Chapter 4 — The 10 Best Questions to Assess a Doctor After Your First Consultation

Consumers' Checkbook. "Medical Advice: Is Your Doctor Measuring Up?" www.checkbook.org/cgi-bin/memberonly/tips/medical_advice. (Subscription required.)

Geehr, Edward C. "5 Questions to Ask When Looking for a New Doctor." *LifeScript.* www.lifescript.com/Health/Everyday/Health_Basics/5_Questions_ to_Ask_When_Looking_for_a_New_Doctor.aspx.

Randa, Jackie. "How to Choose a Good Doctor." *Desert Dispatch.* (Barstow, CA.) www.desertdispatch.com/common/printer/view.php?db=desertdispatch&id =764.

U.S. Department of Health & Human Services, Agency for Healthcare Research and Quality. "Questions Are the Answer." www.ahrq.gov/questionsaretheanswer.

Chapter 5 — The 10 Best Questions When Getting a Second Opinion

Consumers' Checkbook. "Keeping an Eye on Medicare's Impact on Choice of Physicians." www.checkbook.org. (Subscription required.)

Consumers' Checkbook. "Medical Advice—Is Your Doctor Measuring Up?" www .checkbook.org (Subscription required.)

The Eldercare Team. "Getting a Second Opinion." www.eldercareteam.com/ resources/articles/secondopinion.htm.

National Fibromyalgia Association. "When the Orchestra Lacks Harmony, Bring in a Team." www.fmaware.org/site/News2?page=NewsArticle&id=5945.

Thaler, Richard H., and Cass R. Sunstein. *Nudge: Improving Decisions About Health, Wealth, and Happiness.* New Haven: Yale University Press, 2008.

Chapter 6 — The 10 Best Questions for Wellness Checkups

American Diabetes Association. "All About Diabetes." www.diabetes.org/about -diabetes.jsp.

American Heart Association. "Cholesterol." www.americanheart.org/presenter .jhtml?identifier=1516.

American Heart Association. "Lifestyle and Risk Reduction." www.americanheart .org/presenter.jhtml?identifier=3004354#Smoking.

American Lung Association. "Quit Smoking." www.lungusa.org/site/pp.asp?c=dv LUK9O0E&b=33484.

British Heart Foundation. "Family History." www.bhf.org.uk/keeping_your_ heart_healthy/preventing_heart_disease/family_history.aspx.

Centers for Disease Control and Prevention. "Defining Overweight and Obesity." www.cdc.gov/nccdphp/dnpa/obesity/defining.htm.

MedlinePlus. "Cholesterol." www.nlm.nih.gov/medlineplus/cholesterol.html.

National Heart Lung and Blood Institute. "What Is High Blood Pressure?" www .nhlbi.nih.gov/health/dci/Diseases/Hbp/HBP_WhatIs.html.

Chapter 7 — The 10 Best Questions for Men with Fibromyalgia

ChronicFatigueSupport.com. "Overwhelming Evidence Legitimizes Fibromyalgia Pain." www.chronicfatiguesupport.com/library/showarticle.cfm/id/7600.

DrugBank. "Search Term: Fibromyalgia." www.drugbank.ca.

Gulf War Veteran Resource Page. "Forums." www.gulfweb.org/fusetalk.

National Fibromyalgia Association. "The Evolving FM Experience." www .fmaware.org/site/News2?page=NewsArticle&id=5317.

National Fibromyalgia Association. "It's a Guy Thing: Men with Fibromyalgia." www.fmaware.org/site/News2?page=NewsArticle&id=6032.

National Fibromyalgia Association. "Living Life with Hope." www.fmaware.org/ site/News2?page=NewsArticle&id=5315.

National Fibromyalgia Association. "Not Lazy—Not Crazy." www.fmaware.org/ site/News2?page=NewsArticle&id=5316.

National Fibromyalgia Association. "Those Who Can't Do . . ." www.fmaware .org/site/News2?page=NewsArticle&id=5313.

Yahoo Health Groups. "FibroMen Support Group." http://groups.yahoo.com/group/FibroMenSupportGroup.

Chapter 8 — The 10 Best Questions About Fibromyalgia Medications

About.com. "How is Fibromyalgia Treated?" http://arthritis.about.com/od/fibromyalgia/a/fibrotreatment_2.htm.

American Pharmacists Association. "Pharmacy and You." www.pharmacyandyou.org.

Australian Rheumatology Association. "Patient Information: Medicine Information Sheets." www.rheumatology.org.au/community/PatientMedicineInformation.asp.

U.S. Food and Drug Administration. "Recalls, Market Withdrawals and Safety Alerts." www.fda.gov/opacom/7alerts.html.

National Council on Patient Information and Education. "Make Notes and Take Notes: Helpful Steps to Avoid Medication Errors." www.talkaboutrx.org/assocdocs/TASK/269/make_notes.pdf.

Chapter 9 — The 10 Best Questions for Choosing Alternative Therapies for Fibromyalgia

American Pain Foundation. "Complementary/Alternative Medicine Articles & Web Links. www.painfoundation.org/page.asp?file=Links/CAM.htm.

Bassman, Lynette. *The Feel-Good Guide to Fibromyalgia & Chronic Fatigue Syndrome: A Comprehensive Resource for Recovery.* Oakland, CA: New Harbinger Publications, 2007.

Fibromyalgia Information Foundation. "Herbal Medications." www.myalgia.com/Treatment/herbal_medications_carol_burckha.htm.

Mayo Clinic. "Fibromyalgia: Alternative Medicine." www.mayoclinic.com/health/fibromyalgia/DS00079/DSECTION=alternative-medicine.

National Center for Complementary and Alternative Medicine. "What Is CAM?" http://nccam.nih.gov/health/whatiscam.

National Fibromyalgia Association. "Thoughts on a New Integrative Approach." www.fmaware.org/site/News2?page=NewsArticle&id=5233.

Partners Against Pain. "Pain and Integrative Medicine." www.partnersagainstpain.com/professional-medicine/professional-medicine.aspx?id=4.

Teitelbaum, Jacob. *From Fatigued to Fantastic!*, 3rd ed. New York: Avery, 2007.

Chapter 10 — The 10 Best Questions to Avoid Being Scammed

American Board of Medical Specialties. "Online Physician Ratings: Proceed with

Caution." www.abms.org/News_and_Events/Media_Newsroom/Releases/release_
PhysiciansRatings_06_11_08.aspx.

U.S. Food and Drug Administration. "The Facts About Weight Loss Products and
Programs." www.cfsan.fda.gov/~dms/wgtloss.html.

Chapter 11 — The 10 Best Questions Before Participating in a Clinical Trial

CenterWatch. "Background Information on Clinical Research." www.centerwatch
.com/patient/backgrnd.html.

CenterWatch. "Informed Consent: A Guide to the Risks and Benefits of
Volunteering for Clinical Trials." www.centerwatch.com/patient/ifcn_00
.html.

CenterWatch. "Trial Listings by Medical Areas." www.centerwatch.com/patient/
trials.html.

Clinical TrialFinder.com. "Home Page." www.clinicaltrialfinder.com.

Clinical Trial Network. "Potential Participants." www.clinicaltrialnetwork.com/
potential_participants.php.

ProHealth. ImmuneSupport.com. "Fibromyalgia & Chronic Fatigue Syndrome
Clinical Trials." www.immunesupport.com/community/clinical-trials.cfm.

Wikipedia. "Clinical trial." http://en.wikipedia.org/wiki/clinical_trial.

Chapter 12 — The 10 Best Questions to Find a Great Massage Therapist

Associated Bodywork & Massage Professionals. "Fact Sheet." www.massagetherapy
.com/_content/images/Media/Factsheet1.pdf.

Associated Bodywork & Massage Professionals. "To Find a Practitioner." www
.massagetherapy.com/home/index.php.

Massage Health Therapy. "Massage Therapy." www.massagehealththerapy.com.

Natural Healers. "Trigger Point Schools." www.naturalhealers.com/feat-trigger
-point.shtml.

Wikipedia. "Massage." http://en.wikipedia.org/wiki/Massage.

YouTube.com. "Medical Massage For Fibromyalgia." www.youtube.com/
watch?v=ntV_0m5tRLM.

Chapter 13 — The 10 Best Questions for Choosing a Top Acupuncturist

Accreditation Commission for Acupuncture and Oriental Medicine. "Accredited
& Candidate Schools." www.acaom.org/accdtd_cndtdschls.htm.

Acupuncture.com. "A Brief Introduction." www.acupuncture.com/education/
theory/acuintro.htm.

Acupuncture.com.au. "Discussion Forum." www.acupuncture.com.au/forum.

British Acupuncture Council. "Welcome." www.acupuncture.org.uk.

National Fibromyalgia Association. "Contradictory Study Results: Is Acupuncture

Beneficial for FM, Or Not?" www.fmaware.org/site/News2?page=News Article&id=5065.

National Fibromyalgia Association. "The Yin and Yang of Fibromyalgia Syndrome: Treatments Based on the Ancient Wisdom of Traditional Chinese Medicine." www.fmaware.org/site/News2?page=NewsArticle&id=5901.

Wikipedia. "Acupuncture." http://en.wikipedia.org/wiki/Acupuncture.

Chapter 14 — The 10 Best Questions to Get a Good Night's Sleep

About.com. "Sleep Disorders." http://sleepdisorders.about.com.

Fibromyalgia Network. "Sleep Disorders in Fibromyalgia." www.fmnetnews.com/basics-overlap.php#SleepDisorder.

Lundeberg, Thomas and Iréne Lund. "Did 'The Princess on the Pea' Suffer from Fibromyalgia Syndrome?" *Acupuncture in Medicine.* Northwich: 2007. Vol. 25, Issue 4, 184.

National Sleep Foundation. "Fibromyalgia." www.sleepfoundation.org/site/apps/nlnet/content2.aspx?c=huIXKjM0I xF&b=2450839&ct=3500567.

National Sleep Foundation. "Sleeping Smart." www.sleepfoundation.org/site/c .huIXKjM0IxF/b.4381259.

The Pain Clinic. "Sleep." www.painclinic.org/aboutpain-sleep.htm.

SleepNet. "Sleep Disorder Sites." www.sleepnet.com/links.htm#sleep4.

WebMD. "Sleep Disorders Health Center." www.webmd.com/sleep-disorders/default.htm.

Wikipedia. "Sleep disorder." http://en.wikipedia.org/wiki/Sleep_disorder.

Chapter 15 — The 10 Best Questions to Tame Your Stress

Fibromyalgia Information Foundation. "Deep Relaxation Techniques." www .myalgia.com/Treatment/connie2.htm.

Fibromyalgia Information Foundation. "From Herbert Benson's Mind Body Institute." www.myalgia.com/Treatment/herbert_benson.htm.

Joffe, Rosalind. *Women, Work, and Autoimmune Disease—Keep Working, Girlfriend!* New York: Demos Medical Publishing, 2008.

Maslach, Christina, and Michael P. Leiter. *The Truth About Burnout: How Organizations Cause Personal Stress and What to Do About It.* Hoboken, NJ: Jossey-Bass, 1997.

Chapter 16 — The 10 Best Questions to Lose Weight and Eat Well

Fibromyalgia Network. "Diet and Exercise." www.fmnetnews.com/resources -daily-exercise.php.

Lorigan, Janice. *High Fructose Corn Syrup and the Fibromyalgia Connection: Fibromyalgia Recovery Handbook.* Bloomington, IN: AuthorHouse, 2007.

Moeller, Mary, and Joe M. Elrod. *The Fibromyalgia Nutrition Guide*. Pleasant Grove, UT: Woodland Publishing, 1999.

Rawlings, Deirdre. *Food that Helps Win the Battle Against Fibromyalgia: Ease Everyday Pain and Fight Fatigue*. Beverly, MA: Fair Winds Press, 2008.

Smith, Shelley Ann. *Fibromyalgia Cookbook: More Than 120 Easy and Delicious Recipes*. Nashville, TN: Cumberland House Publishing, 2002.

Chapter 17 — The 10 Best Questions to Find a Great Gym or Fitness Club

AARP. "Choosing a Health & Fitness Club." www.aarpfitness.com/articles .aspx?articleID=1005.

American Council on Exercise. "Before You Start an Exercise Program." www .acefitness.org/fitfacts/fitfacts_display.aspx?itemid=94.

Dryland, David, and Lorie List. *The Fibromyalgia Solution: A Breakthrough Approach to Heal Your Body and Take Back Your Life*. New York: Warner Books, 2007.

familydoctor.org. "Fibromyalgia and Exercise." http://familydoctor.org/online/ famdocen/home/common/pain/tr eatment/061.html.

International Council on Active Aging. "How to Select an Age-Friendly Fitness Facility." www.icaa.cc/facilitylocator/ICAA%20Facility%20Test.pdf.

Mayo Clinic. "Fitness." www.mayoclinic.com/health/fitness/SM99999.

Medical Fitness Association. *The Medical Fitness Model: Facility Standards and Guidelines*. Medical Fitness Association: Richmond, VA: 2008.

Official Journal of American College of Sports Medicine. "Physical Activity and Public Health in Older Adults: Recommendations." www.acsm.org/AM/Text Template.cfm?Section=Home_Page&Template=/CM/ContentDisplay.cfm& ContentID=7789.

Chapter 18 — The 10 Best Questions to Hire a Top Personal Trainer

The American Council on Exercise. "Exercise and Fibromyalgia." www.acefitness .org/fitfacts/pdfs/fitfacts/itemid_89.pdf.

familydoctor.org. "Fibromyalgia and Exercise." http://familydoctor.org/online/ famdocen/home/common/pain/treatment/061.html.

Fibromyalgia Exercise. "What You Can Do." http://fibromyalgiaexercise.net.

Fibromyalgia Information Foundation. "Exercise Advice." www.myalgia.com/ Exercise%20advice.htm.

International Council on Active Aging. "Exercise and Chronic Pain." www .myalgia.com/Exercise/ICAA_Functionalu_Vol4_1.pdf.

MyFibro.com. "Fibromyalgia Exercise." www.myfibro.com/fibromyalgia-exercise.

Staud, Ronald, and Christine Adamec. "Exercising, Losing Weight, and Avoiding

Trigger Foods/Drinks." In *Fibromyalgia for Dummies*. New York: Wiley Publishing, 2002.

Chapter 19 — The 10 Best Questions for Your Emotional Health After Fibromyalgia

AboutCom. "Coping with Fibromyalgia & Chronic Fatigue Syndrome." http:// chronicfatigue.about.com/od/copingwithfmscfs/a/coping.htm.

Borysenko, Joan. *Minding the Body, Mending the Mind,* rev. ed. New York: Da Capo Press, 2007.

CFIDS & Fibromyalgia Self-Help. "Emotions." www.cfidsselfhelp.org/archive_emotions.htm.

Mayo Clinic. "Fibromyalgia pain: Create a Plan for Coping." www.mayoclinic .com/print/fibromyalgia-pain/AR00055/METHOD=print.

National Fibromyalgia Association. "How Psychotherapy Can Help FM-Related Depression." www.fmaware.org/site/News2?page=NewsArticle&id=6235.

National Fibromyalgia Association. "Maintaining a Positive Attitude: Ten Strategies." www.fmaware.org/site/News2?page=NewsArticle&id=5340.

Selfridge, Nancy, and Franklynn Peterson. "Cut Old Angers Down to Size." *In Freedom from Fibromyalgia: The 5-Week Program Proven to Conquer Pain*. New York: Three Rivers Press, 2001.

Chapter 20 — The 10 Best Questions When Talking with Your Partner About Fibromyalgia

Fibromyalgia Network. "Relationships Supplement." www.fmnetnews.com/ resources-daily-relationships.php.

National Fibromyalgia Association. "Living with a Loved One with Chronic Illness: An Interview with Gregg Piburn." www.fmaware.org/site/News2?page =NewsArticle&id=5353.

Skelly, Mari, Kelley Blewster, and Devin J. Starlanyl. *Women Living with Fibromyalgia*. Alameda, Calif.: Hunter House, 2001.

Vanderzalm, Lynn. *Finding Strength in Weakness*. Grand Rapids, MI: Zondervan Publishing, 1995.

Well Spouse Association. "Home Page." www.wellspouse.org.

Williamson, Miryam E., and Mary Anne Saathoff. "Committed Relationships." In *The Fibromyalgia Relief Book: 213 Ideas for Improving Your Quality of Life*. New York: Walker & Co., 1998.

Chapter 21 — The 10 Best Questions About Sex, Intimacy, and Fibromyalgia

About.com. "Sexuality and Disability Myths and Facts." http://sexuality.about .com/od/disability/p/disability_sex1.htm.

Marek, Claudia Craig. "Keeping Your Relationships Alive." In *The First Year: Fibromyalgia: An Essential Guide for the Newly Diagnosed.* New York: Avalon Publishing, 2003.

National Fibromyalgia Association. "Ouch! Don't Touch Me!" www.fmaware.org/site/News2?page=NewsArticle&id=5339.

WebMD. "Pain Management: Maintaining Intimacy." www.webmd.com/pain-management/pain-management-maintaining-intimacy.

Chapter 22—The 10 Best Questions Before Talking with Your Children About Fibromyalgia

Halpern, Susan P. "Talking to Children About Illness and Death." In *The Etiquette of Illness: What to Say When You Can't Find the Words.* New York: Bloomsbury, 2004.

Kids in Crisis. "Welcome." (Online help for teens.) www.kidsincrisis-website.org/content/publish/default.shtml.

"Parents and Grandparents: Getting the Most Out of Your Time." *Fibromyalgia Network Journal.* July 2008, 14.

Remen, Rachel Naomi. *Kitchen Table Wisdom.* New York: Penguin Group, 2006.

Rainbows. "Welcome." (Online grief and loss resources for children of all ages.) www.rainbows.org.

Wallace, Daniel J., and Janice Brock Wallace. *Fibromyalgia: An Essential Guide for Patients and Their Families.* New York: Oxford University Press, 2003.

Chapter 23—The 10 Best Questions to Decide About Telling Others

Berne, Katrina, Robert M. Bennett, and Daniel L. Peterson. "Relationships." In *Chronic Fatigue Syndrome, Fibromyalgia, and Other Invisible Illnesses.* Alameda, CA: Hunter House, 2001.

The Lubbock Avalanche-Journal. "Patients Battle Perception of Fibromyalgia." www.lubbockonline.com/stories/052208/hea_281647018.shtml.

McGinnis, Alan Loy. *The Friendship Factor: How to Get Closer to the People You Care For.* Minneapolis, MN: Augsburg Fortress Publishers, 2004.

Paul, Marla. *The Friendship Crisis: Finding, Making, and Keeping Friends When You're Not a Kid Anymore.* New York: Rodale Books, 2004.

Women and Fibromyalgia. "Fibromyalgia and Friendships." http://womenandfibromyalgia.com/2008/07/25/fibromyalgia-and-friendships.

Chapter 24—The 10 Best Questions Before Joining a Support Group

Arthritis Foundation. "Local Office Directory." www.arthritis.org/chaptermap.php.

Fibromyalgia Association UK. "Support Groups." www.fibromyalgia-association uk.org/content/view/16/47.

FM-CFS Canada. "FM & CFS/M.E. Support Groups." www.fm-cfs.ca/support .html.

HealthyPlace.com. "Sympathy-Seekers Invade Internet Support Groups." www .healthyplace.com/site/article_faking.asp.

National Fibromyalgia Association. "Support Group Leaders Newsletter." www .fmaware.org/site/PageServer?pagename=community_fameSupportConnection Newsletter.

Open Directory Project. Fibromyalgia: Support Groups." www.dmoz.org/Health/ Conditions_and_Diseases/Musculoskeletal_Disorders/Connective_Tissue/ Fibromyalgia/Support_Groups.

ProHealth's ImmuneSupport.com. "Support Group Related Sites." (Provides links.) www.immunesupport.com/community/category.cfm?cat=Support%20Group.

PsychCentral. "What to Look for in Quality Online Support Groups." http:// psychcentral.com/archives/support_groups.htm.

Schiff, Harriet Sarnoff. *The Support Group Manual: A Session-By-Session Guide.* New York: Penguin Books, 1996.

Schwarz, Roger. *The Skilled Facilitator,* 2nd ed. San Francisco: Jossey-Bass, 2002.

Chapter 25 — The 10 Best Questions for Financial Health After Fibromyalgia

American College of Rheumatology. "Patient Assistance Programs for Rheumatology-Related Drugs." www.rheumatology.org/public/acrast.asp?aud =pat.

American Pain Foundation. "Financial Issues." www.painfoundation.org/page .asp?file=documents/doc_017.htm.

Centers for Medicare & Medicaid Services. "Medicare Prescription Drug Coverage." www.medicare.gov.

NeedyMeds.com. "Home Page." www.needymeds.com.

Partnership for Prescription Assistance. "Partnership for Prescription Assistance." https://www.pparx.org/Intro.php.

Chapter 26 — The 10 Worst Questions to Ask Someone with Fibromyalgia

Guilmartin, Nance. *Healing Conversations: What to Say When You Don't Know What to Say.* San Francisco: Jossey-Bass, 2006.

Jones, Sue. *Parting the Fog: The Personal Side of Fibromyalgia/Chronic Fatigue Syndrome.* Reading, KS: LaMont Publishing, 2001.

Wooten, Patty. Jest for the Health of It. "Articles by Patty Wooten." www .jesthealth.com/frame-articles.html.

Chapter 27 — The 10 Best Questions for Your Spiritual Health and Fibromyalgia

Association of Professional Chaplains. "Healing Spirit." (Newsletter.) www .professionalchaplains.org/index.aspx?id=678.

Canfield, Jack, Mark Victor Hansen, and Heather McNamara. *Chicken Soup for the Unsinkable Soul: 101 Stories.* Deerfield Beach, FL: Health Communications, 1999.

Dagwood, N. J., ed. *The Koran.* New York: Penguin, 2004.

Duke University: Center for Spirituality, Theology and Health. "Research and Publications." www.dukespiritualityandhealth.org/publications.

Holy Bible, King James Version. Peabody, MA: Hendrickson Publishers, 2004.

Institute for the Study of Health and Illness. "Finding Meaning in Medicine." www.meaninginmedicine.org/home.html.

Spirituality & Health. "Articles." www.spirituality-health.com/spirit/content/ articles.

Tzu, Lao. *Tao Te Ching: A New English Version.* New York: Harper, 2006.

University of Florida Center for Spirituality and Health. "Bibliographies." www .spiritualityandhealth.ufl.edu/bibliographies.

Wikipedia. "Spirituality." http://en.wikipedia.org/wiki/Spirituality.

Young, Caroline, and Cyndie Koopsen. *Spirituality, Health and Healing.* Sudbury, MA: Jones and Barlett Publishers, 2005.

Meet the Experts

The author interviewed each of the following experts for this book.

Rebecca Allison, M.D., FACC, FACP, is an experienced cardiologist in Phoenix, Arizona, the president-elect for the Gay and Lesbian Medical Association, and chair of the American Medical Association's advisory committee on gay and lesbian issues. Dr. Allison has been chosen by her peers as one of Phoenix Magazine's "Top Doctors in Phoenix" for several years.

Stephen Barrett, M.D., a retired psychiatrist and consumer advocate in Allentown, Pennsylvania, is best known for his popular Web site, Quackwatch, a nonprofit organization whose mission is to "combat health-related frauds, myths, fads, fallacies, and misconduct." His Web site is www.quackwatch.org.

Brent A. Bauer, M.D., is the director of the Complementary and Integrative Medicine Program at the Mayo Clinic in Rochester, Minnesota. Board certified in internal medicine, Dr. Bauer is an associate professor of medicine at the Mayo Medical School and featured in the DVD, *Mayo Clinic Wellness Solutions for Fibromyalgia* (2007).

Hamilton Beazley, Ph.D., is the scholar-in-residence at St. Edward's University in Austin, Texas, and the author of *No Regrets: A Ten-Step Program for Living in the Present and Leaving the Past Behind.* Dr. Beazley has been interviewed on *Oprah,* NBC, CNN, and many other television and radio shows and networks. The Web site is www.stedwards.edu.

Martha Beck, Ph.D., is a writer and life coach pioneer who specializes in "life design" by helping people design satisfying and meaningful life experiences. Dr. Beck has lived with fibromyalgia for almost thirty years. She overcame its extreme challenges to earn three degrees from Harvard University, write dozens of bestselling books and articles, and to become a columnist for the *Oprah Magazine.* Her latest book is called *Steering by Starlight* and her Web site is www.marthabeck.com.

Herbert Benson, M.D., is a world-renowned pioneer in mind-body medicine, director emeritus of the Benson-Henry Institute for Mind Body Medicine at

Massachusetts General Hospital, and a former Harvard University professor. Dr. Benson has written more than 180 scientific publications and eleven books, including the best seller *The Relaxation Response* (1975). His institute's Web site is www.mbmi.org and his Wikipedia entry is at http://en.wikipedia.org/wiki/Herbert_Benson.

Norman Berk is a certified financial planner, CPA, personal financial specialist, and J.D. He founded Professional Asset Strategies, LLC, a fee-only financial firm in Birmingham, Alabama. Both he and his wife are cancer survivors and activists. His Web site is http://proassetsllc.com.

Kathy Berra, MSN, NP-C, FAAN is the clinical director of the Stanford Heart Network for online cardiovascular health assessment and education. She has over thirty-five years in cardiac care and is the past president of the American Association of Cardiovascular and Pulmonary Rehabilitation and the Preventive Cardiovascular Nurses Association. Her organization's Web site is www.stanford/heart.net.

Lorraine Biros, LCPC, is the director for client services and a licensed clinical professional counselor at the Mautner Project: The National Lesbian Health Organization in Washington, D.C. Ms. Biros has more than twenty-eight years of counseling experience in the lesbian and gay community. The organization's Web site is www.mautnerproject.org.

Jessica Black, ND, is a naturopathic physician in private practice in McMinnville and Portland, Oregon, and author of the book, *The Anti-Inflammation Diet and Recipe Book.* Dr. Black specializes in complementary therapies, pediatrics, and women's medicine including natural hormone balancing. Her Web site is www.afamilyhealingcenter.com.

William Blatt, M.P.H., is the manager of tobacco control programs at the American Lung Association National Headquarters and oversees all of the Association's tobacco prevention and cessation programs. He was responsible for the 2007 edition of the adult cessation program, Freedom From Smoking, and is supervising the creation of the 2009 edition of the youth cessation program, Not On Tobacco®. His organization's Web site is www.lungusa.org.

Peter Block has an international reputation as a management consultant and as the author of best-selling books, including *Flawless Consulting: A Guide to Getting Your Expertise Used* and *The Answer to How Is Yes,* a book that examines the underlying assumptions about asking questions. His newest book is *Community: The Structure of Belonging,* and his Web site is www.peterblock.com.

M. K. Brennan, MS, R.N., LMBT, NCTMB, ACMA, is a North Carolina massage therapist in private practice and a hospital nurse case manager. She is currently the president of the American Massage Therapy Association (AMTA) and has been an active AMTA volunteer since 1993. Ms. Brennan is published in various publications including the *Journal of Bodywork and Movement Therapies*.

Charles R. Cantor, M.D., DABSM, is a neurologist specializing in the diagnosis and treatment of sleep disorders. He is the medical director of the Penn Sleep Centers of the University of Pennsylvania Health System and a clinical associate professor of neurology and medicine. Dr. Cantor was recognized by *Best Doctors in America* during 2005–2006 and 2007–2008. The Web site is www.pennhealth.com.

Barbara (Bobbi) P. Clarke, Ph.D., RD, is a professor and codirector for the University of Tennessee's Center for Community Health Literacy. She has more than thirty years of experience in public health education and community development and leads a Tennessee-wide community health literacy program. The program's Web site is http://fcs.tennessee.edu/healthsafety/phealth.htm.

Daniel J. Clauw, M.D., is a professor of anesthesiology and medicine in the University of Michigan's Division of Rheumatology, the director of the Chronic Pain and Fatigue Research Center, and director of the Michigan Institute for Clinical and Health Research. An early pioneer in fibromyalgia research, Dr. Clauw leads a multidisciplinary team studying effective treatments. The Web site is www.med.umich.edu/painresearch and this group contributed heavily to www.knowfibro.com.

Harriette Cole reaches a broad multiethnic audience with her nationally syndicated advice column *Sense and Sensitivity*. Ms. Cole is a creative director of *Ebony* magazine, heads Harriette Cole Productions, and coaches recording artists including notable musicians such as JoJo, Alicia Keys, and Mary J. Blige. Her Web site is www.harriettecole.com and her Wikipedia entry is at http://en.wikipedia.org/wiki/Harriette_Cole.

Caldwell B. Esselstyn, Jr., M.D., is a clinician and author of the best-selling book *Prevent and Reverse Heart Disease*. Since 1968 he has been associated with the Cleveland Heart Clinic, including as staff president. Dr. Esselstyn was awarded the Benjamin Spock Award for Compassion in Medicine and has published over 150 scientific papers. His Web site is www.heartattackproof.com.

Betty Ferrell, RN, Ph.D., FAAN, is a clinician and research scientist in pain management at City of Hope National Medical Center in Duarte, California. She has been in nursing for more than thirty years and focuses on spirituality issues, quality of life, and palliative care. Dr. Ferrell is a Fellow of the American Academy of Nursing and has authored over 270 publications including five books on pain management and nursing care. The Web site is www .cityofhope.org/Pages/default.aspx.

Edwin B. Fisher, Ph.D., is a professor in the Department of Health Behavior and Health Education in the School of Public Health at the University of North Carolina at Chapel Hill. He is also global director of the American Academy of Family Physicians Foundation's project, *Peers for Progress,* an international program to promote peer support for diabetes management. For more than twenty-five years, Dr. Fisher has been a leading expert, researcher, and international contributor to smoking cessation efforts. He is widely published, including the books *7 Steps to a Smoke Free Life* (1998) and *How to Quit Smoking Without Gaining Weight* (2004).

Daniel Forman, M.D., is an assistant professor of medicine at the Harvard Medical School and the director of the Exercise Testing Laboratory and Cardiac Rehabilitation at the Brigham and Women's Hospital in Boston. He is also a staff physician at the Geriatric Research, Education and Clinical Care Center for the Veterans Administration. Dr. Forman has done extensive research on cardiovascular disease and preventive lifestyle modifications.

Rachael Freed, MSW, LICSW, LMFT, has practiced psychotherapy for thirty years, founded Women's Legacies, and authored several books for well spouses including *Heartmates: A Guide for the Spouse and Family of the Heart Patient,* 3rd ed. (2002). Ms. Freed is also a senior fellow at the University of Minnesota's Center for Spirituality and Healing. Her Web sites are www.Heartmates.com and www.womenslegacies.com.

Mark Gorkin, MSW, LICSW, is a licensed clinical social worker who calls himself "The Stress Doc." Mr. Gorkin is a motivational speaker, humorist, organizational consultant, and the author of two books on stress management. His Web site is www.stressdoc.com.

Dorothy (Dot) Gerecke, R.N., FCNA, is a former nurse living in Horsham, Australia, who struggled for ten years before being diagnosed with fibromyalgia in 1992. Born and raised on a farm in Tasmania, Australia, Ms. Gerecke attended nursing school and practiced nursing in obstetrics, intensive care, and coronary care. She is active with various online fibromyalgia support groups in Australia and the United States.

John Gray, Ph.D., is the world's number-one-selling relationship author. An international gender and relationship expert, his *New York Times* best-selling *Men Are from Mars, Women Are from Venus* books have sold more than thirty million copies worldwide. Dr. Gray's latest book, *Why Mars and Venus Collide,* is available at www.marsvenus.com/collide and his Wikipedia entry is at http://en.wikipedia.org/wiki/John_Gray_(U.S._author).

Mimi Guarneri, M.D., FACC, is the medical director of the Scripps Center for Integrative Medicine in La Jolla, California. Dr. Guarneri has authored numerous professional articles and the book *The Heart Speaks: A Cardiologist Reveals the Secret Language of Healing.* The Web site is www.scripps.org/locations/scripps-clinic/services/integrative-medicine_integrative-medicine.

Tess Hahn, Licensed Acupuncturist, OMD, Diplomate. Ac. (NCCAOM), earned her Doctorate of Oriental Medicine at California's SAMRA University after training in California and China. She has practiced acupuncture and Oriental Medicine since 1984, served on the Idaho State Board of Acupuncture, and received the Governor's Award for Distinguished Public Service. She is currently the Chair of the Board of the National Certification Commission for Acupuncture and Oriental Medicine. The Web site is www.nccaom.org.

Rosie Hamlin was the songwriter and lead singer of the 1960s recording group Rosie & the Originals, best known for their 4 million-selling hit song, "Angel Baby," one of Beatle John Lennon's favorite songs. Diagnosed with fibromyalgia in 2000 and currently living in New Mexico, Ms. Hamlin previously shared her personal story through a 2005 National Fibromyalgia Association's conference and *AWARE* article. Her Web site is http://rosieandtheoriginals .com and her Wikipedia entry is at http://en.wikipedia.org/wiki/Rosie_ Hamlin.

Larry F. Hamm, Ph.D., FAACVPR, FACSM, is the current president of the American Association of Cardiovascular and Pulmonary Rehabilitation and director of the Clinical Exercise Physiology Program at The George Washington University Medical Center in Washington, D.C. He is certified by the American College of Sports Medicine as a program director for exercise programs. The Web site is www.aacvpr.org.

David J. Hanson, Ph.D., is a professor emeritus of sociology at the State University of New York at Potsdam and an international expert on alcohol consumption. Dr. Hanson has written more than three hundred publications, studied alcohol consumption for forty years, and appeared on many national television and radio programs. His Web site is www2.potsdam.edu/hansondj and his Wikipedia entry is http://en.wikipedia.org/wiki/David_J._Hanson.

Julia R. Heiman, Ph.D., is the director of the famous Kinsey Institute for Research in Sex, Gender and Reproduction at Indiana University in Bloomington, Indiana. For more than sixty years the Kinsey Institute has been the worldwide leader in studying human sexuality, gender, and reproduction research. The Web site is www.kinseyinstitute.org.

Peggy Jensen, RD, MBA, has more than twenty-five years as a registered dietitian, including work in New York City developing a "cardiac prudent diet" for her cardiac patients. Ms. Jensen also coordinated a nutritional educational program for the American Heart Association on heart healthy foods. Ms. Jensen owns a nutrition consulting business and teaches school in Virginia.

Kim Dupree Jones, R.N., FNP, Ph.D., is an associate professor in the Schools of Nursing and Medicine at Oregon Health & Science University in Portland, Oregon. She leads several major fibromyalgia research studies and has authored nearly one hundred publications. Dr. Jones maintains a clinical practice specializing in fibromyalgia and is the current president of the Fibromyalgia Information Foundation. The Web site is www.myalgia.com.

Sharon Jordan-Evans, president of the Jordan Evans Group, is a speaker, certified executive coach, and workplace consultant. She is also the coauthor of two best-selling books on workplace issues: *Love 'Em or Lose 'Em: Getting Good People to Stay* and *Love It, Don't Leave It: 26 Ways to Get What You Want at Work.* Her Web site is www.jeg.org.

Richard Koonce is president of Richard Koonce Productions, Inc., a human resources consulting and communications firm in Brookline, Massachusetts. Mr. Koonce is an experienced writer, consultant, facilitator, coach, and interviewer and has authored four business books. His Web site is www.richard koonce.com.

C. Everett Koop, M.D., was the U.S. Surgeon General from 1982 to 1989. He is the recipient of numerous awards, including seventeen honorary doctorate degrees and the Presidential Medal of Freedom. Still going strong at ninety-plus years old, Dr. Koop stays current with medical education and patient care issues. During his tenure as a high-profile Surgeon General and throughout his long career, Dr. Koop has been an outspoken advocate for improving patient-physician communications. His Wikipedia biography is at http://en.wikipedia .org/wiki/C._Everett_Koop.

Dorothy Leeds, MA, is an internationally acclaimed best-selling author, trainer, keynoter, sales consultant, and expert in questioning skills. Known as the "Questioning Crusader," she has written 12 books including *The 7 Powers of Questions* (2000). Her media exposure includes NBC's *Today* show, ABC's *Good Morning America,* and the *New York Times.* Ms. Leeds also appears in Broadway shows. Her Web site is www.dorothyleeds.com.

Abby D. MacLean is an information systems engineer specializing in security and information assurance for the nonprofit MITRE Corporation in Virginia. She works with U.S. federal government agencies to help them find solutions to challenging and modernization problems. Ms. MacLean was diagnosed with fibromyalgia in 1993. Her organization's Web site is www.mitre.org.

Anna Maravelas, Licensed Psychologist, MA, is an international consultant specializing in stress and conflict in the workplace. She is the author of *How to Reduce Workplace Conflict and Stress* (2005) and the founder of TheraRising, Inc., in St. Paul, Minnesota. Ms. Maravelas's work has appeared in the *New York Times, Forbes, O: The Oprah Magazine,* and *Harvard Management Update.* Her Web site is http://therarising.com.

Lynne Matallana, president and cofounder of the National Fibromyalgia Association, became so ill in 1993 with chronic pain and disturbed sleep that she became bedridden. Over the next two years, she went to thirty-seven doctors before being diagnosed with fibromyalgia. Based on her personal experience, Ms. Matallana has created an organization that is an educational and networking powerhouse for empowering people with fibromyalgia and educating the medical community. The Web site is www.fmaware.org.

Cicily Carson Maton is a certified financial planner and the founder of Aequus Wealth Management Resources, a Chicago-based financial planning and investment firm that specializes in advising people during major life transitions. She has appeared several times on the television show, *Right on the Money.* Her Web site is www.aequuswealth.com.

Michael McNett, M.D., is the owner and medical director of the Center for Fibromyalgia, Fatigue, and Chronic Pain. He specializes in treating fibromyalgia and chronic pain patients and is considered a top researcher and thought leader in this field. Dr. McNett coauthored the book, *The Everything Health Guide to Fibromyalgia: Professional Advice to Help You Make It Through the Day* (2006). The Web site is www.cffcp.com.

Rear Admiral Kenneth P. Moritsugu, M.D., M.P.H., retired in 2007 as the acting U.S. Surgeon General in Washington, D.C. Admiral Moritsugu's forty years in public health service included many honors, such as his service as Deputy Surgeon General for nearly ten years. Admiral Moritsugu's Wikipedia biography is at http://en.wikipedia.org/wiki/Kenneth_P._Moritsugu.

Debbie Nigro is an award-winning radio personality, champion of women, author, speaker, and business executive based in New York. Ms. Nigro has interviewed hundreds of people for her radio shows, which are aired in 450 markets. Her Web site is www.firstwivesworld.com.

Scott Peck, Ph.D., and Shannon Peck of San Diego, California, cofounded

TheLoveCenter, an educational organization dedicated to raising relationship and spiritual awareness, and have coauthored several books. Their Web site is www.thelovecenter.com.

Gregg Piburn is a management consultant and author of the book *Beyond Chaos: One Man's Journey Alongside His Chronically Ill Wife* (1999) about the impact of his wife's fibromyalgia on their relationship. He frequently gives presentations on their experiences to others touched by chronic illness. Mr. Piburn and his wife, Sherrie, who live in Loveland, Colorado, speak nationally about their experiences. His Web site is www.leadersedgeconsulting.com.

Christina M. Puchalski, M.D., directs the Institute for Spirituality and Health (GWish), is an associate professor of medicine at The George Washington University in Washington, D.C., and is a practicing physician. Dr. Puchalski is recognized for pioneering the integration of spirituality and health care and has authored the book *A Time for Listening and Caring: Spirituality and the Care of the Chronically Ill and Dying.* The Web site is www.gwish.org.

Linda Pütz, MA, is a career and life coach in Frederick, Maryland, and has two teenaged sons. Despite her diagnosis of fibromyalgia ten years ago, she runs her own business, LKP Assessment and Development Systems, which is dedicated to making winning matches between organizations and individuals. Ms. Pütz is a certified life purpose coach and has a master's degree in counseling. Her Web site is www.yourtalent.org.

Vicki Rackner, M.D., is a board-certified surgeon who left the operating room to help patients, patients' families, and caregivers partner more effectively with their doctors through her company, Medical Bridges. She is also an author, speaker, and consultant, including coauthor of *Chicken Soup for the Soul: Healthy Living Series* books and several patient self-help books. Her Web site is www .medicalbridges.com.

Susan Sikora hosts a television talk show in San Francisco, California, and has interviewed hundreds of political, entertainment, and health celebrities. Ms. Sikora is an Emmy winner who formerly hosted live talk shows for PBS, CBS, NBC, and ABC. The Web site is http://cwbayarea.com.

William Sonnemaker, MS, PES, CES, CSCS, is the CEO of Catalyst Fitness and an award-winning personal trainer including IDEA's 2007 International Personal Trainer of the Year, National Academy of Sports Medicine 2007 Pursuit of Excellence winner, and Atlanta's Best Trainer since 2005. His many credentials include professional certification from the American College of Sports Medicine. His Web site is www.fitnesscatalyst.com.

Devin J. Starlanyl is an internationally known expert on fibromyalgia, the author of two popular fibromyalgia books, *Fibromyalgia and Chronic Myofascial Pain: A Survival Manual,* 2nd ed. (2001) and *The Fibromyalgia Advocate* (1999), and has fibromyalgia herself. Ms. Starlanyl has also authored numerous other related publications and presents seminars in the U.S. and abroad. Her Web site is www.sover.net/~devstar.

Richard Stoltz, Ph.D., CAPT, USN, has been a mental health professional for over thirty years. During his twenty-two years in the navy he has served in numerous administrative and clinical capacities. He currently serves as the assistant chief of staff at the U.S. Navy's Bureau of Medicine and Surgery.

H. Robert Superko, M.D., FACC, FAHA, FACSM, is the executive director of the Center for Genomics and Human Health at St. Joseph's Translational Research Institute in Atlanta. His background includes numerous research projects and scientific publications. Dr. Superko wrote the book, *Before the Heart Attacks,* to help explain detailed aspects of heart disease risk factors. The Web site is www.stjosephsatlanta.org.

Helen Thomas is a legendary question asker, news service reporter, columnist, and member of the White House press corps. She served for almost sixty years as a correspondent and White House bureau chief for United Press International, challenging every president since President Kennedy with questions from her front-row seat during press conferences. Ms. Thomas's Wikipedia biography is at http://en.wikipedia.org/wiki/Helen_Thomas.

Paige Waehner is a personal trainer certified through the American Council on Exercise, a freelance writer, and has more than thirteen years of exercise experience. She trains her Chicago clients at home as well as online at Plus One Active. Ms. Waehner authored the book *About.com Guide to Getting in Shape* among other publications. Her Web site is http://exercise.about.com.

Kim Allan Williams, M.D., FACC, is an expert in clinical and nuclear cardiology and the 2008 board chairperson for the Association of Black Cardiologists. He also serves on the Board of Trustees of the American College of Cardiology and the American Board of Internal Medicine (Cardiovascular Diseases). Dr. Williams was voted one of Chicago's top doctors in 1996, 2000, 2004, and 2007. His organization's Web site is www.uchospitals.edu.

Cary Wing, Ed.D., is the executive director of the Medical Fitness Association, dedicated to defining industry standards of excellence for medical fitness centers. Dr. Wing has more than twenty-five years of experience in the health and wellness field, and gives frequent presentations on women's health issues. Her organization's Web site is www.medicalfitness.org.

Patrick B. Wood, M.D., is chief medical officer of Angler Biomedical Technolo-

gies, LLC, a private company whose primary focus is improving the understanding and treatment of fibromyalgia. He formerly directed the Fibromyalgia
Care Clinic at LSU Health Science Center in Shreveport, Louisiana. Recognized by the National Institutes of Health for his innovative research,
Dr. Wood is the originator of the dopamine theory of fibromyalgia. He also
serves as a senior medical advisor to the National Fibromyalgia Association and
presents at global scientific conferences. His organization's Web site is www
.lifebeyondpain.com/index.shtml.

Patty Wooten, R.N., BSN, has nearly forty years of experience in nursing. After
witnessing firsthand the power of therapeutic humor, she created an educa-
tional/consulting company in Santa Cruz, California, called Jest for the
Health of It. Ms. Wooten has entertained audiences around the world and is a
veteran of countless radio shows, television shows, and print media, including
NBC's *Real Life* and *USA Today.* Her Web site is www.jesthealth.com.

Paul Yurachek, J.D., CPA, is a certified financial planner, and a senior financial
advisor with Gurtz, Yurachek and Associates, a financial advisory practice of
Ameriprise Financial Services in Bethesda, Maryland. Mr. Yurachek is a former employee of the Internal Revenue Service and specializes in retirement
planning, tax planning, and estate planning.

Index

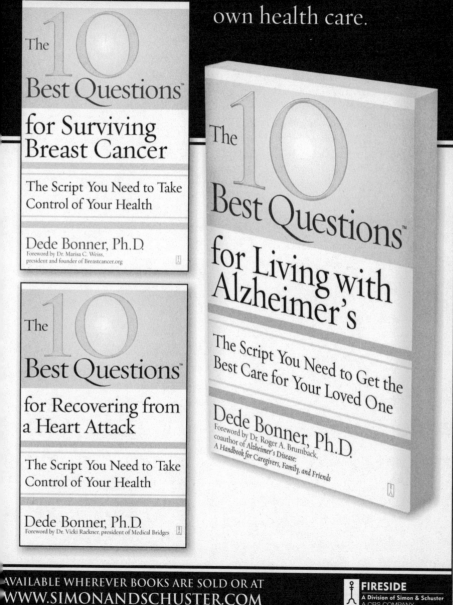